# Lose Weight
# Naturally

## JD Lovil

Lose Weight Naturally

Copyright © 2015 J D Lovil.

ALL RIGHTS RESERVED

Published 2015 by JD Lovil Publishing

ISBN-13: 978-1517577889

ISBN-10: 1517577888

# Disclaimer

This book is intended to be a source of information to begin or continue your pursuit weight reduction and health. It is not an authoritative work by a professional in any health or psychological field, and should not be taken as such.

The Author has concepts that have some bearing on the subject matter, and he thinks that they may be useful for the interested party seeking a change, but all ideas presented should be taken only for consideration. The reader should decide the value of such ideas for themselves.

The Author does not present an opinion of any other techniques or ideas used by any other persons dealing with the subject. The Reader should make an evaluation, and as always, he or she should always apply due skepticism to this and all other ideas presented.

# CONTENTS

# INTRODUCTION

**Many** people in the modern world find themselves overweight. They will spend years imitating a Yo-Yo. They try first one diet and then another, attempting to get rid of the extra pounds. None of these frantic efforts seem to work.

Many of these diets are unbalanced nutrition. It is obvious that an unbalanced diet will cause you to gain weight. The organism that you will eat indiscriminately, as you seek the missing nutrients.

If one wants to lose weight, one must first eat fewer calories. You do this by having everything the body seeks in the fewest calories of food. Most diets do not address the major causes of overeating at all, other than a token nod toward an exercise routine.

**LOSING WEIGHT NATURALLY** will address the parts of life not addressed by the other guys. This book is a whole life approach to losing weight. As such, it is as applicable to any other life issues you might have as it applies to a weight issue. We will address goals, philosophy, and spiritual categories of life in the process.

.

# 1: THE PROBLEM

**If** you are reading this book, you have been struggling with a weight problem, or a similar quandary, and you are hoping to find a solution to your issue at hand. This book will not be a simple diet book. It will be a whole life makeover, treating those parts of your life that cause the weight complications, and giving you a much happier life.

If you examine your life carefully, you will find that there is not just one reason why you have a weight issue, there are dozens. To change your body, you must change many of your activities, your consumptions, and the image you carry around in your head of who you are.

You can find the reasons for this dilemma in many categories of your lifestyle. The amount and quality of your sleep is a big factor. What you eat, and how you eat it are vital to weight. The stress level you have and the types of stress you have are other areas of vital importance.

Everyone knows that exercise is important in the weight-loss regime but did you know that not all exercises are created equal? You may walk, or play sports hit the gym or work at a physically strenuous job. You might just ride herd on your pets or the rug rats. Each of these activities carries their emotional packages, and fit the needs of your body in different ways. It is important that you use the right mix of these activities to maintain or reduce your weight.

Let us continue to discuss in brief what the problems are, but in the order that we will be discussing them in detail in the rest of this book. It is important to realize that the categories of activities and areas of concern are not black and white. Stress and exercise are frequently extremely interconnected, and the same applies to most of the categories and areas discussed in this book, so in some cases, the Reader may think that the definitions are a bit arbitrary. The Reader would be right, but you have to slice the pie somehow, right?

The first issue to address is the problem of stress. It is important to understand that there are good stress situations, and there are bad stress situations. Stress is a necessary behavioral response to certain situations, and we all have certain types of stressful situations that cause us to grow and accomplish wonderful things, and other areas of stress that can only harm us. The trick is to allow the first kind of stress, avoid the second kind, and learn not to carry any of the stress around with us all the time.

What you eat and drink is obviously very important to your health and weight. It is only one factor to address, and most Dieters will begin and end their efforts to lose weight with this one factor. Even this activity will be poorly planned and executed, mostly due to the morass of bad information about what the human body needs to consume, to be healthy and of proper weight. It is not usually the Dieter's fault. They are following bad advice, addressing only one of the areas of their life that they need to change, and when they lose focus, they will yo-yo right back to their original over-weight condition.

Bad learned behaviors and habits can be a real obstacle. You know the sort of habits I mean. When you are young, your parents taught you that candy was a reward and that veggies were a punishment that you had to eat before you could eat the good stuff. Most of us can also remember the Adults that ladled out way too much food on our plates, and admonished us to clean our plates.

Assuming that the previous issues do not turn your crank, you may have a problem with emotional issues. Some of the standard ones are those involving confrontations, or those dealing with interaction with people. You might get nervous about taking a test or dealing with any number of events that are important to you. You also may be avoiding other people, either physically, or socially. You may be a wallflower at every social gathering, or do as I did when I was young; slip out the back door as they came in the front door, and go fishing. These reactions may or may not be because of a Self-Image problem.

One of the most important and least appreciated health needs is for a consistent string of good night's sleep. A large part of your metabolic activity and up to 95% of your healing takes place only when you are asleep. You cannot cheat on this one. If your body and mind need eight hours of uninterrupted sleep, getting six hours means that you are slowly degrading your health. Your body's default low energy setting is to store fat, so not enough sleep will tend to put the pounds on you.

Your self-image is the way you see yourself. It is primarily a composite of your Self-Esteem, your Self-Confidence, and an actual visual image of you that you represent yourself with when you think about You. A three-hundred-pound muscle bound prizefighter could lose a fight with a 120-pound accountant if he has a self-image that believes that he cannot win the fight. A bad self-image may cause you to pack on weight if you think that you are a loser at whatever is important to you, and getting chubby is a nifty way to be out of the running.

One last issue is the icing on the cake. You may not be an utter victim of any of the previous problems as described, although I suspect that to some degree, you have fallen victim to more than one of them. Even without any of these as explicit difficulties, you may be growing more and more depressed because you see your life as going nowhere. This Self-Esteem based depression will tend to make over-eating seem a very attractive alternative to worrying about spinning your wheels and getting nowhere.

The odd thing about our wonderful academic facilities is that they are great at giving us the tools to solve life's problems, but they are not so good at telling us how to use them. Having all of the tools you need to reach your goals does not help you very much if you never learned to set those goals properly. It is like starting out on a trip without knowing where you are trying to go, and even without a map.

The next chapter will deal with all the ins and outs of the sort of stress that will cause you a weight problem, and the chapter after that will deal with how to deal with stress properly.

.

# 2: ALL ABOUT STRESS

## Bad Stress

**There** is a variety of stresses that you will encounter every day. Stress can cause anger, depression, and fear and will sometimes result in responses that are far greater than called for in the circumstances. You will frequently try to avoid the stressful situation or the people associated with that situation. We built the fishing industry on the need to avoid the stresses and dramas of life, but there are far better reasons to fish than to avoid the bad scenes.

A lot of us grow up thinking of ourselves as not measuring up to what other people might expect of us. Some of the things we imagine are that they do not think that we are smart enough, or ambitious enough, or pretty enough, or in the case of weight issues, we are either too thin or too fat. Most of that is probably not true, and we forget that most people just do not care about us unless we are in some way important in their lives.

If we think of ourselves as inadequate in some of these ways, we will tend to interact with other people with a certain amount of fear and trepidation, dealing with others from a position of non-confidence and weakness. One reason that we are concerned so much with other people's opinions is that our social instincts are operating in a strange alien environment. Let me explain.

Humans developed over a long period to be social animals. Up until the last few centuries, humans lived in very small communities composed of fifty to a couple of hundred people, most of which would be related to each other to some degree. Strangers were potential enemies, and everyone that we knew, we could expect to be dependent on, in one situation or another. In our modern world, we are not allowed to treat strangers as enemies in the traditional way, so our unconscious minds lump them into the category of 'fellow villagers,' and we treat them as part of our community if we have to interact with them. Most of the time, we ignore the extraneous people in our life with whom we do not have to interact. Think about the typical New Yorker's reaction to people around them in distress.

In our historic communities, if you interacted with other people without killing them, they were your comrades, and you *did* need to measure up to what they thought you needed to be. If you were not fast enough, clever enough, or strong enough, you could get them killed, in an interaction with them. We carry that relationship with us into our modern world, and then we apply the same life or death importance to other people's opinions of us in a situation where it is not really appropriate.

Let us say that you are twenty pounds overweight. Unless you plan to have a sexual relationship with the persons you encounter, what difference does it make what their opinion of your weight is? If it bugs you, you should at least consider finding a beach where nobody knows you, putting on that tiny bikini, and let your freak flag fly! If you were a Dude instead of a Dudette, I would prefer to see a pair of trunks on you instead.

The most frequent method of dealing with social stress is to do poorly in communicating, inversely proportional to how much is at stake in the circumstances for you. You may feel sexually attracted to the person with whom you are speaking. In this case, you may miscommunicate, using inappropriate body language, speech nuances, and even verbiage to sabotage your chances of getting what you want out of the conversation. At the extremes, you will not communicate at all, act as the proverbial Wallflower, or even leave via the back door.

The social situations that we evolved to deal with were much simpler than those that our modern world contains. We would kill, drive away, or arrange a marriage with strangers. We would defend, assist, and protect our fellows. We would forage for an hour of so each day for food in the nearby forests, and sit in the shade or play in the water in the heat of the day. Other than a leader for the occasional hunt or warfare expedition, nobody was your superior in your activities. It was not until Chiefs started becoming Kings that there was someone around authorized to tell us what to do. Bosses are not natural.

The current work environments, even the touchy-feely ones, are not natural for us either. Our bosses make us want to pick up a big club and make our points, and the drudgery and repetition of the typical job make us want to walk into traffic. Modern work is not a natural concept. In the 1800s, the white Landowners in Hawaii used to get very upset when they would talk the natives into doing the hard work. The Hawaiians would spend a couple of hours making a playful attempt to complete the work tasks, and then the owners would find that they had run away to play at the beach.

When Human genetics cannot cope with an environment, we do an amazing thing. When we go to school, or to work, or we fight a modern war, we create and wear another personality, which is better suited to deal with that environment. This Persona is partially consciously, and mostly unconsciously, designed and created by our minds to cope more successfully with the problems we might encounter. If you think carefully, you will realize that your behavior at work is very different to the way you behave at home, or in other situations. A soldier is built to survive the stresses of the modern battlefield by both traditional training procedures, and by unconscious adaptation to the realities of a soldier's life.

Wearing your nifty Work Persona, you are much better able to deal with that abusive Boss or the sheer boredom and frustrations of the daily grind. The problem is that the newly created Persona is seldom a perfect fit for the environment, and sometimes we find it hard to take it off when we get home. Sometimes, the insane demands of the Boss are beyond any reasonable ability to cope with, regardless of your modifications. Sometimes, we spend a few minutes when we get home dealing with the rug rats as though they are our minions. In both cases, the tension created is hard to get rid of, and the temptation to get the cake and ice-cream out to deal with it can be overwhelming.

I have noted with a certain amount of amusement that our poor excuse for health reporting touts a change of women's health as a mystery. A long time ago, women were mostly involved with taking care of the house and kiddies, and the man would go out into the world to make money for her to spend. In recent years, women have begun to complete advanced degrees, and they have entered the workforce in droves. I think that we can all agree that these are good things.

The problem with the modern condition is that in the history of Mankind, women have done the traditional nurturing thing in the cave, hut, or house until recently. This adaptation to a nurturing but boring set of tasks creates a lifestyle that would cause the average man to pull out his hair and cut his throat. Over time and natural selection, women have come to be able to deal with these specific stresses well, and they did not derive a lot of damage from the stresses they experienced. You might say that, for women, this is a kind of good stress. The result was that women tended to live longer than their male counterparts did.

Now women are entering into the same work-a-day world that has been shortening the men's lives. The women are finding that they are dying earlier from the same stress-related diseases of heart attack and stroke that the men have been dying from all along. Welcome aboard, women! You are now equal to men in all things, including the right to an early death.

Women may have an even harder problem dealing with work-related stress than men have, due to the typical ways that women unwind from stressful situations. Women have always been the social glue in human societies. They developed the need to talk among themselves to get a certain level of validation of their feelings, and this made them feel better, and also served the useful function of creating a communications hub for the community. When it is bad news, we call it gossip. Whatever, most women feel the need to talk about their day until they feel validated, and finally they can calm down.

Men usually have a different way of unwinding. They sink into their favorite chair, and turn on the television, with a beer in hand. Alternatively, maybe they go straight to their workshop. Whatever they do, the last thing they want to talk about is work. Usually, they do not want to talk at all. Give a man his preferred unwind environment, and he is mostly de-stressed from work in about twenty minutes. The woman is still talking herself down two hours later.

The World of Survival selected different social functions for men and women. The man or woman that could not adequately deal with the stresses of living in history usually did not live, and so both learned behaviors and genetics developed to deal with specific types of stress for which they were selected. Work is not a natural environment, but men have a few centuries more than women have had to adapt to that world.

One of the biggest stresses in life is finances. Most of us live paycheck to paycheck, and it does not make us calm to realize that our political leaders do not understand that the majority of their constituents would be on the streets, if what they do interrupts the economic flow. We fret and worry about where we can find the money for dentists and braces, school, rent, automobiles and a million other things we need.

Most of us have little or no ability to save money for a future emergency. It is not natural to horde an inadequate supply of anything. In the natural world, if there is only a small amount of food available, it is more valuable to stuff yourself than it is to put it aside to rot. When you cross the desert, you will survive better if you drink your water as desired until it is gone. Rationing it out will kill you quicker.

Our natures do not equip us to save, but we are smart enough to stress about it when we do not save. I do not think I need to ramble on about the stress of money worries. Everyone knows someone who had committed suicide because of lack of money.

The final sort of stress that I will discuss is the stress that derives from competition. Competing in a sport or game can be a lot of fun, but when the stakes are personal, competition can cause a huge amount of stress. You can lose that promotion, lose that court case, or get a divorce. All of these things can cause a huge amount of stress with the loss of a wife or husband, kids, having to watch as the half of your holdings you still control are not sufficient to sustain the business or home or lifestyle that you had. Stress is all about potential loss.

These are only a few examples of competition stress. Anytime you are in a situation, and you feel that sour ball of discomfort in the pit of your stomach, the chances are good that some aspect of competition stress is responsible. The convolutions of this sort of stress are endless, and it is present in almost all of the other stressor situations. I will leave it at that for you to mull over.

In the next section, we will examine the various sorts of stress that are good for you. Bet you did not see that coming!

## Good Stress

Stress is a natural process. It has its uses, and it can be beneficial to the person that has it. It is an emotional and physical state that either prepares the body for the fight or flight modes, or the process of tensing up the muscles preparing for the same modes causes it.

Just because stress exists does not mean that it has to cause permanent damage. The maintaining of the stressful state too long by the body causes the damage, usually long after any possible use that you may have for the stress reaction. In most cases, if the stressful state is brief, followed by a successful resolution of the situation, it causes no damage and may *actually* contribute to the health of the individual.

If you meet someone that you would like to have a relationship with, you will probably feel a certain amount of stress, until you see that your attempt to begin a relationship is being successful. Once the situation resolves to your satisfaction, you will feel a rush of the body's natural morphine, also known as endorphins, and a glow of cozy, intimate feeling brought on by a naturally produced hormone called oxytocin. All of the bad effects of stress are behind you, and the body is rewarding you for a job well done. If you can maintain the endorphin and oxytocin state, you will live longer and be happy.

You cause the same sort of condition when you ride the Ferris Wheel, Free Climb, Bungee Jump, parachute or any of the other activities that 'Adrenaline Junkies' generally engage in, except that they don't usually get the oxytocin, just the endorphins. I am not certain if a serial killer gets both chemicals when they make a successful kill, and I am not sure that I want to know.

Any activity that gives you the warm glow of success at the end of it, and where the stress state does not last indefinitely can be a healthy activity. Even in the rare times, when you are hard at work in your job, you realize that you just made a wonderful goal happen. In short order, the other minions and even the Overlords will come to you and give you the accolades that you deserve, and you will experience healthy stress.

Most Entrepreneurs work harder and longer than any employee, making their dream business come true. They are acting on their own initiative, and when they succeed, they will feel the unmitigated glow of success. No matter how hard they work, they feel like they are playing the most interesting game in the world. That, as they say, makes all the difference.

The play is the key, and there are two different ways to do it. Some sorts of play are hard and stressful at the moment, but the player sees the success or failure of the game to be of no true importance. To others, they are seeking success, but every portion of the game completed provides the glow they seek. Even if they reach the goal, it is only the next step in the game. The game only ends when they take that final dirt nap.

One of the reasons that many people love playing computerized games is because the success or failure of the game playing is not important to them. In a second, they can restart the game. I noticed long ago that while I was a very good pool player, I could never play the game for money. If there were nothing important riding on the outcome, I would play a very good game. Should I bet on the game, it was a certainty that I would 'choke' on my shots. The same problem was noticeable with taking tests. I realized long ago that I could ace almost any test I took, as long as it was not important to me how I did. If it was important, it was a lot harder to ace it.

I noticed the same phenomena when I was in my dating heyday. The less I cared about the relationship I was getting into, the easier it was to engage in it or to replace it with another opportunity as desired. The lesson to be learned here is simple. When you are involved in completing a task or activity, the less you worry about the successful completion of it, while maintaining the efforts, the better your outcome will be.

This is a process created by the person's Self-Esteem, that wonderful inheritance that we all get from the adults in our childhood experiences. Most of us have some damage of our Self-Esteem, and we have to create workarounds until we can find ways to do some repairs. We will cover that subject in a later chapter, along with both temporary and permanent fixes for the problem.

Most types of play involve creating wonderful structures or systems, either mentally or physically. This can be in the form of campaigns, buildings, businesses or anything else that can be a pattern that the person can create and develop. This can be playing a game, building a business, inventing a device, solving a mathematical problem, or accomplishing any goal that you may have.

It is important to note that any life that has a proper handle on the healthy way to deal with stress is one that is relatively happy. It is also true that, for the person to be happy, he cannot be just whiling away the days of his life. The happy person is always active, creating and building something that they enjoy doing.

The person must have a set of goals that they are acting to complete to be happily active. To complete the goals successfully, they must be written down and before you act upon the goals. We will discuss the making and completion of goals in detail in a later chapter.

I know that some of you may have started to worry that this book would never get to things that had a direct connection to your diet, and how to lose weight. Fear not, the next chapter deals with what we do wrong in our diet, and how to eat properly. Prepare to be amazed, amused, and gruntled.

# 3: ALL ABOUT EATING

## The Overview

**Humans** are omnivores. Of all the animals on this planet, humans and pigs may have the most versatile digestive systems that exist. The digestive needs of the two species are almost identical. A time-honored method of checking unknown foods for suitability is to feed it to a hog. If the hog eats it, it is okay for people as well.

We are well equipped for finding food in a land where food is a scarce commodity. We have instincts that drive us to gorge ourselves when food is plentiful, preparing for the famine that will surely come. We were never designed to live in a world where food is available in endless supply, such as the world we live in today. Surviving in the Land of Plenty requires a plan.

## Bad Eating

A variety of factors contributes to gaining and maintaining a bad fat to lean ratio. Some of these are obvious. Some of these factors are not so obvious as simply overeating. Consuming a lot more calories of food than you need for your activity level is one of the obvious reasons for gaining weight. The reasons we do this may be less obvious.

Our digestive systems are complex and intricate systems for getting and using nutrients that our body needs to build itself, act as fuel for our activities, and heal any damages that we may have inflicted upon us. Factors that determine the outcome of eating includes eating habits, the ratio of needed nutrients to proteins, carbohydrates, and fats in our diets, intestinal flora populations and our mental processes and self-images that we hold.

One of the newest discoveries regarding obesity is that the types and quantities of intestinal flora (The bacteria that lives in our guts) determine largely how much and what part we digest of what we eat. These species of bacteria live in our guts symbiotically. They are a major part of our digestive process, breaking down what we eat into smaller bits that our bodies can absorb and use. For that service, they get to live inside us, and nibble on everything we eat. Without them, our digestive system would not work, and we would waste away.

The bacteria in our bodies outnumber human cells ten times. We are 90% bacteria and only 10% human. This is a sobering thought, isn't it? Which bacteria are in our guts makes a big difference on whether we turn the food we eat into energy to do our thing, or stored as fat, usually in the bikini area. Misuse of antibiotics and the presence of antibacterial substances in the environment and the body cause the flora populations to change into a fat producing configuration that you really do not want.

One of the newer problems for intestinal bacteria is genetically modified foods. Some of the newer GMOs include a high tolerance for insecticides, which also kills many kinds of bacteria as well, and some even produce their own insecticides, which will collapse bacteria populations, also. I believe, that one day soon, we will discover proof that the 'hive collapse' syndrome, happening now to bees, will be because of anti-insect substances inherent in the GMO pollen sources, which the bees tap to make their honey.

Our systems include a hunger response mechanism, in part adjusted by the bacteria present. If the species that turns the hunger pangs off is not present, you will feel hunger even when you are full. If the diet that we eat lacks in certain key nutrients, such as some of the minerals our body needs, we will eat more of the food available, under the theory that if you eat enough, eventually you will get enough of the missing nutrients from the diet. Depleted soil makes depleted food, and getting enough of the right nutrients by eating larger meals is not always possible in today's world.

In an ideal world, the food you eat will contain everything it should contain, and you will not have to overeat to get all the nutrients your body needs. Unfortunately, poor forestry and agricultural practices have served to leach the trace, but vital nutrients out of the soil, and so the food we eat rarely has the minerals our bodies need to function correctly. If you still need a vital trace mineral after eating a full meal, the meal will not entirely satisfy your hunger impulses, and you will almost certainly overeat, as you seek to consume enough of that vital nutrient.

One of the reasons that some people overeat, and gain unwanted weight, is an absurdly simple habit. Somewhere in our inherited behaviors, we tend to eat fast, to avoid the possibility that someone or something will take our meals away from us. This is a real problem because our hunger triggers only turn off our hunger response when the digestive system has time to digest some of the consumed food, and time to establish that we have eaten the needed nutrients, and then it turns off the 'Hunger' sign. If you eat too fast, you over-eat. It is as simple as that.

When I was a young beanpole, I watched, as my sister would wolf down a big meal as fast as possible. She also spent her life on endless diets. She would never listen to me when I told her that she should slow down, chew each bite slowly, and stop when she felt full. I know that people will not act on advice 99% of the time, but really, that was dumb!

When people are trying to sell you a new diet, almost invariably it will be a very lopsided diet. It will push you to eat almost exclusively protein, or carbohydrates, or fat! It never occurs to those people that you eat to get the nifty little nutrients that you need, so if you eat all protein, you are starving your body for the nutrients that plants will provide. If your diet avoids animal protein, you will try to keep eating until you get enough usable proteins in your diet, and that means you will keep eating and getting fat.

The problem with a Vegan diet is that, while the amino acids needed are present to make proteins, your body likes to start with some animal protein, not amino acids. This means that a Vegan diet starves your body for proteins, and keeps you hungry. Just because everything is present in your diet does not mean that it is in a form your body can use.

One of the problems with diet is that it varies a bit among populations. Asians usually get more food value out of rice than Caucasians do. Eskimos can eat 98% fat in their diets, but the rest of us would have a problem with that diet. Native Americans (Indians to the rest of us) will stay healthy on traditional foods, but they get fat on hamburgers. We all adjust to what was available to our bloodlines, over time, but a few things touted about our dietary needs are absolutely in the lie category.

The foods that were historically available to your ancestors determine your nutritional needs. We should consider two parts of this history. First, the mineral mix required by your body to function correctly is approximately the same as the ratio that was found in the seawater approximately five hundred million years ago. The other part is the mix of vitamins and proteins, fats, carbohydrates and other constituents that have been available in the diets of our ancestral forms. The longer our ancestors ate the foods, the better we are adapted to using them.

Minerals originally present in the soil of new land formed by upraising, or by volcanic formation, began to be leached into the oceans by dissolving in rainwater and flowing into the oceans. This has led to mineral poor soils, and commercial fertilizing usually only replaces a small portion of the missing minerals, such as nitrates and calcium, in the form of lime. In previous centuries, forest fires and chimney ashes would wind up in the soil, replacing some of the depleted minerals with minerals brought up into the trees by deep root systems.

In our own species' history, our ancestors ate what they could find, or what they could catch. They ate small game, insects, eatable plants, eggs, mollusks, fish, and small amounts of grain as the major sources of food. Big game, milk, and large sources of grain were rare treats. More recently, populations have started to digest large quantities of agricultural products such as grains and milk in higher quantities.

## Good Diet

The FDA has always had some version of the so-called 'Food Pyramid,' which purports to tell us what we should eat as its version of a healthy diet. It has always given the largest portion of the structure to grains and vegetables, with a good portion of dairy products, and the smallest portions go with meats, fats, and sugars.

The Food Pyramid was obviously designed for the health and welfare of some alien creature. It is certainly not a suitable diet for humans. Eating large quantities of grains or milk products is not a diet for which most of humanity is adapted to eat. More people have allergies to these foods than in any other food groups because of this. Let me break that down a little.

My ancestry is in large part Northern European, with a significant smattering of American Indian, and probably tiny amounts of every other population. My European ancestry makes me able to eat oatmeal, rye and other grains that have been eaten in Northern Europe for several hundred years without a significant problem. I like rice, but it is like eating air. Corn is a great food for me as well. I can drink milk without problems.

Most Asians can eat rice, and they will get the same good benefits from it that I do from oatmeal. Many people from Asia and Africa have big problems with milk products. What we tolerate as food is dependent on how long our ancestors have been eating it. Most people have no problem eating meat, because meat is a long-standing food source, and because it is a semiperfect match for the ingredients of our body. Eggs come in a close second.

Meat is the perfect food because it contains everything we have in our bodies. Our ancestors ate insects and small game for a long time, and so, these are the best meat sources for us to eat. Red meat is good on rare occasions, but it can be a real problem if you overeat it.

Therefore, you should eat only a little grain that suits your particular ancestry, small game such as rabbit, insects if you can stomach the idea, fruits, and vegetables. This brings us to the so-called Paleo Diet. I have seen some odd foods listed as Paleo meals, but it is a good idea of how you should eat.

In recent years, the Paleo Diet has become popular. It features most of the common vegetables, meats, and eggs, and stays away from some of the worst of the current fads. Think substitute cornbread for white bread, small game, and fish. A Paleo Diet resembles the meals that your Grandmother used to make, a lot more than it does a McDonald's meal. Some of the websites that tout the Paleo Diet include foods with more starches and grains than is natural and healthy, but even they are much better for you than fast foods.

Let us review some of the things that will form a proper human diet in today's world. You need to eat foods relatively high in protein and fats, such as meat, preferably small game, fish, and bird meat. You need to eat a variety of green leafy vegetables, fruits and starch sources such as potatoes, or one of the alternatives. You should eat only small amounts of grains, of the types that your ancestry adapted to eating. Drink or eat only the level of Milk products that your body can tolerate. Mushrooms are an excellent food to add to your diet. Just do not pick wild mushrooms yourself. Even experts can pick the wrong ones.

You should eat all food very slowly, and only eat small portions at any one time. Your food grows in soil depleted of many of the 90 important minerals. You should supplement your food with a mineral supplement. This will keep you from overeating to obtain enough of these minerals.

Maintain yourself in a calm state. Your body releases hormones if you are stressed that promote overeating. Stress eating usually will turn into fat rather than muscle or energy if strenuous activity does not immediately follow the stress.

Your body is designed to function with low amounts of food available, so eat slowly, and stop eating as soon as the hunger signals go away. Filling your stomach the rest of the way up is not necessary.

# 4: HABITS AND BEHAVIOR

## Background Information:

**We** are all instructed and conditioned by the actions and words of the Adults in our life as young children. We imitate their behavior. We listen to everything they say. We do things to solve our childish problems. If what we do works, we repeat the same actions. Eventually, the actions that we repeat, because they worked for us, become a habit.

We form our personalities as children. Our successful habitual actions, our experiences, and the things told us as true, form those personalities. Our personalities are nothing more than the set of behaviors that our minds have formed to be successful in seeking and securing those things we need, and the Self-Image that we form from these behaviors and our beliefs.

Drug addicts are typical of the formation of habits and behaviors around the process of securing and taking the drugs to which they have become addicted. Meth addicts sample the drug in the beginning, and they love the effects of energy, euphoria and perhaps even the social nuances. They want to repeat the experience. Seeking out the drug and using it becomes a habit that rapidly becomes a set activity. The personality is modified by this habit, as the behavior associated with the experience of securing and using the drug becomes a large part of the personality of the drug user.

In the following paragraphs, we will usually refer to the habit aspect of this activity, but you should assume that we will also address the behaviors where appropriate. It is rarely clear where habits end, and behavior begins.

## Bad Habits:

As a young Lad or Lass, you were doubtlessly admonished to "clean your plate." You may also have been clearly rewarded for a job well done with candy or some other sweet treat. As you hit puberty, you may have felt yourself to be unattractive, and decided that if you cannot win, why should you play the game of dating. You can just keep eating until the subject of dating goes away. After all, three hundred pounds of bouncing love is much less likely to have to decide on loving.

We are also evolved to live in a world with never enough to eat. In that world, you have a good chance of losing the food you did not eat to someone who is bigger and stronger. We now name them Bullies, but they still would be eating your food instead of you. This means you have a built-in instinct to eat your food fast so that you get to keep it.

We create our habits from our experience of what actions we have taken in the past that worked, our beliefs, our self-image, and what others told is true in our formative years. The more times our habits succeed in getting us what we want, the stronger those habits become. At some point, the habits we develop become a central part of our personality, and even when they cease to work, we still maintain them, because they have become part of who we are.

One of the habits that will illustrate this is cigarette smoking. Early on, smokers pick up the habit, because someone influential in their lives smokes. Smoking serves a number of purposes in the Smoker's life, and these are the next anchor points to the habit. Let us elaborate on the values that the act of smoking gives to the Smoker.

Smoking is a valuable reason to take a break from work or some other onerous task. It provides nicotine to the body, a useful precursor to a needed neurotransmitter, which energizes the brain, and to some extent the body. The activity has a calming effect on the Smoker. Smoking serves as a versatile social tool in awkward situations. The act of smoking is a body-language level bonding activity between Smokers.

These are all value-added assets to the Smoker. Of course, the over-smoking of cigarettes also contributes to COP and other lung diseases. The Smoker is now considered an untouchable in today's society, and it now costs lots of money. None of these things matter to the Smoker. Smoking has become a part of who he is, and if he gives it up, he will always miss it.

At our core, we all believe that doing the right thing and being successful is the same thing. We think that what we do is right, or we would not do it. We may recognize bad aspects to what we do, but we can justify this because the world is not perfect, and if we succeed in what we do, it must have been the right thing to do.

Everything we do is ultimately for our best interests. If you worship a god, you worship for the good benefits that you think you will receive. You do not worship to benefit the deity. This is true of every action you take. Your habits exist to obtain valuable benefits for you, even if they no longer do so. Smoking may no longer provide the calmness, breaks and clarity it once did, but you feel better when you smoke, so you continue to smoke.

You fulfill your Parents' expectations of you by doing those things in a manner that they would approve. To secure the approval of your spectral parents, you clean your plate. You expect a sweet after you accomplish a task, or if you have been a good boy or girl. You eat and live your life to fulfill your opinion, or your parent's opinion, of how deserving you are of rewards or punishments. We can frequently lie about ourselves in words, but our opinions of ourselves are usually broadcast loud and clear to the world in our body language and our actions.

Some of our habits are because of our self-image. Some of them are deficits due to our focus on other things. Take messiness, for instance. You may have a messy house, because it may reflect your Self-Image, or it may simply be because you are busy doing other things, and you never get around to cleaning up the mess. This is true less often than we may be willing to admit, but it is true, at least some of the time.

There is an old saying that you are either messy in your life, or in your mind, but not in both. I doubt that this is an Eternal Truth, but you do tend to be either an extrovert or an introvert. If you are an extrovert, your focus is in your external world, and having a clean house is probably important to you. If you are an introvert, your focus is internal, and you may be indifferent to the mess in your house.

## Good Habits:

It is fortunate for us that most of these bad habits can be changed or eliminated. Some of the solutions are easy and simple. Some of the solutions are a little more exotic and may take a little time. Like everything else, if you decide to accomplish it, every bad thing you want to get rid of is under your control.

Some of the bad habits can be modified. For instance, cleaning your plate is not that bad. Just make a point of never loading your plate with way more than you should eat, and you are golden. You will need to abolish some bad habits entirely. I do not know if changing your eating speed is a new habit or a modification of an old one. Either way, you should substitute eating slowly for eating fast. After twenty minutes of slow eating, I guarantee that you will feel full.

It is not necessary to avoid sweets. If you choose to see them as a reward, reward yourself with a small treat, if you eat a balanced meal of the Paleo variety. You just change the task that you are rewarding and put the reward into healthy proportions, and it will work for you.

Many of the reasons that you may overeat, or that you are eating a bad diet, is because of your self-image. Your self-image is in large part determined by your beliefs, which define the world you live in, and your place in it, the latter for most people. Your parents foisted many of your beliefs upon you. The good news is that you can change your beliefs.

You should take a pen and paper and make two columns on the paper. In the left column, write down your central beliefs about the world. Do you believe in a god? How does that define who you are? Do you believe that you are worthy of good things, or do you believe that you need punishment? Think about this hard, and write down the truth. Just make sure nobody else reads your writing on this. Keep going until you run out of important things in writing down your beliefs.

To the right of these beliefs you have, write a belief that you think would serve you better. For instance, if you think you deserve punishment; maybe you want to write down that you deserve a reward for the Hero you are, and tweak it into something that will serve you better to believe. Do this for every belief you wrote in the left column unless you think that the current belief is one that serves you well.

Once you have decided on what beliefs that would serve you well to have, list them, and then memorize them. Recite them to yourself every time you feel drawn back into the bad beliefs, and recite them to yourself daily. Once you have them in your mind, start visualizing and entertain fantasies about what your life is like when you believe them. Start living your life according to the new beliefs. Sooner than you think, they will replace your old beliefs, and your life will be far happier and more successful based on the new beliefs. Your self-image will change, and you will see that your body will change along with your self-image.

We will explore this more when we get to the chapter on creating your Persona for your new life. Until then, you can work on incorporating your new beliefs into your life.

You should concentrate on eating a balanced diet, which will emphasize meats and vegetables, and reduce your intake of grains and dairy products to suit your particular body needs. Research your ancestry, to determine what your ancestors ate; which is an important factor in what is healthy for you to eat.

Generally speaking, eat meats, fats, root products like potatoes, turnips, carrots and such, fruits of most sorts, and a small quantity of grains. Eat all the mushrooms you can get, and only the level of dairy products that you can eat or drink without allergic effects, such as mucus discharge or body effects.

I think that most Americans can eat a lot of corn products. Unfortunately, most corn is now GMO, and so may contain pesticides, either made by the plant or absorbed by the corn. Keep that in mind, in case eating corn products cause you to feel worse. Research Paleo diets, and be critical of the obvious biases in the choices that the writer may bring to the table.

The most important factor to bring to the mind of the serial dieters among us is to eat a well-balanced meal, eat it slowly, and stop when you stop feeling hungry.

# 5: EMOTIONS AND SERENITY

## Background:

**Everyone** knows that negative emotions have a bad effect on the body. Stress is the base result of negative emotions, and it figuratively, and sometimes literally, tears the body apart. Stress is the main result of negative emotions such as fear, anger and all the component emotions of depression.

We have already established that stress causes the body to turn the food you consume into fat around your middle. It is the body's way to prepare you to go through some bad times ahead, one of the things that your genetics thinks is the likely result of sustained stress in your life. Evolution thinks that you cannot have long-standing stress unless you are losing the battle; hence, you are losing your hunting grounds or your food source, so it prepares your body to survive the coming lean days.

The opposite effects are true of living with positive emotions. Your genetics think that your world is safe, and the food is plentiful, so it turns your meals into energy to go out and procreate, and play in the sunshine. This means you lose the weight you have, and you continue to have happy days as long as the mean old wolf stays away.

Emotions have a profound effect on the body, including weight. You should cultivate positive emotions, and reduce or eliminate the negative emotions to modify your life in many ways, not just your weight. Live longer, be happier, and be healthier by having a positive emotional state. Alternatively, you can choose to die young, be sick and sad. It is all your choice.

## Bad Emotions:

We all know that stress is bad. Most of the time, we are even correct. Some sorts of stress are good, and we will get to those. Most of the so-called negative emotions, such as anger and fear result in putting stress on us. This is the famous *fight or flight* mechanism, and it is a good thing if the situation calls for you to fight or to run away. Unfortunately, we live in a world where, most of the time, the proper response to the stress causing situation does not call for fighting or running away, so we keep the stress way too long. That feels bad, and it *hurts*.

Prolonged stress is bad stress. It causes diseases, nervous conditions, mental illnesses and promotes weight gain, as the hormones produced prepares your body to survive the foreseeable future by storing nutrients as fat around your torso. To prevent this, you must find a way to be as stress-free as possible. Sometimes, the best thing to do when you feel stress is to engage in some form of vigorous sport. This vigorous activity can sometimes dispel stress in the system that has no obvious target.

Next to eating the proper proportions of the right foods, the most important aspect of your life is to manage your stress level. Most of the other things you can do to lose weight are using various tools to reduce the stress level you experience. The following chapters will detail those tools, and how to use them, and then we will discuss what we have learned to do as a comprehensive process for reducing the weight you seek to lose.

## Good Emotions

The body, to promote a condition of health and welfare of the person, produces good emotions. They engender a healthy system, a clear mind, a longer life and a better shot at securing all those good things that we all want and need, including reproduction.

No normal situation exists in the modern world, where the negative emotional states are more desirable to the person than a positive emotional state. The only circumstance when the negatives have a useful function is when the person is involved in a life and death survival struggle. A ***vigorous running away*** will usually take care of that. You should be running toward a happier situation.

When you are calm, happy and enjoying working towards your goals, you are healthier, slimmer, and more active. When you get a good night's sleep, your social life or family life is better. There is no downside to being happy. You should try it.

One of the biggest and most ignored parts of being happy is to be working toward goals. We will discuss these in a future chapter, but for now, let us discuss the benefits. When you are involved in working toward something you want, you will find that you will concentrate on the mental aspects of the work for long periods. You will feel a deep sense of satisfaction as you complete each part of your goal. You will also find that you feel wonderful while doing these things, and science suggests that this deep concentration causes your life to be extended and less disease prone.

It is an ignored fact that goals are a necessary part of happiness, and maintaining a positive emotional life. It is not enough just to live, for humans; we must also be working toward something important to us. This lack of goals is the biggest flaw in most people's lives.

The tools that you need to build a happier life, and to work on and complete goals are meditation, visualization, writing down and affirming the goals, and the immediate engagement with the working of those goals. Meditation can start out just by closing your eyes and clearing your mind of thoughts. Visualization can start as simple daydreams of what having the goal in hand will be like, affirming the goals can be as simple as writing them down and re-reading them each day, and immediate engagement is putting the next steps on a To-Do list and immediately start working on it. These are not always easy, but they are simple. As you get better at each of these, you can modify them with more advanced forms, but the important part is to get started.

When you are not feeling the bad aspects of bad emotional states, you are getting the good effects that come from the good emotions. A good emotional state is the default setting for human beings, and it is only the inhumane lifestyles to which life subjects us, which put us into the stressful holding patterns that cause our problems.

# 6: THE SLEEP FACTOR

## Background:

**Sleep** is essential to the health and functioning of the individual. It is a must, to get good sleep if you want to maintain your weight and your health within any reasonable parameters. At least 95% of all the healing that your body undergoes takes place only when you are asleep. If you objectively observe your body functions, you may have noticed that wounds just sit there and stare back at you, doing nothing to heal, until you get some sleep. Sleep, and when you wake, you are amazed at the progress the injury has made in healing itself.

There are four major bands of wave frequency put out by the brain during normal activities. The Beta band is the frequency that dominates while you are your nervous, awake self. You experience an Alpha state when you are sitting quietly and calmly, with nothing bothering you. You experience Theta state when you are deeply asleep. During this stage, you have a sense of identity, but it is a dreamy and nebulous state. When you lose that sense of self as a separate entity, you are entering into a Delta state, the state that, among other conditions, is the primary one for coma patients.

The brain always emits all four frequencies. When we say that we are in Alpha state, what we mean is that the Alpha frequency dominates in brain activity at that time. Beta waves are the highest frequency of the four waves, at 40 to 12.5 Hz, with Delta the lowest frequency in the range of 4 down to 0 Hz. Alpha waves are at 13 to 8 Hz, while Theta is 8 to about 4 Hz. In a state of extreme high-energy mental concentration, one may experience a fifth form, the gamma state, above 40 Hz.

The Beta state is associated with the normal waking activity, and Alpha with calm and light meditation states, Theta with high meditation and light to moderate sleep, and Delta with deep sleep, unconsciousness, and loss of self-identifiers.

### Bad Sleep:

People rush through their lives these days. They speed to work in the morning traffic jam at the breakneck speed of five miles per hour of bumper-to-bumper chaos.

They take orders from bosses that they are pretty sure are not smart enough to dress themselves without help in the mornings. After that, it is off to home, to take care of those parasites that await you, which you refer to as your family and pets. Finally, you have put the obligations of the day to bed, along with the last of the family. You only have a limited number of hours available to sleep, before you have to get up and do it all again.

You spent the whole day winding your nerves up tight. Most likely, you will waste half of the available sleep time winding down enough to sleep. By the time you wake up, you are lucky if you were in bed for five hours. You only got about two hours of what your granddad would have called "real sleep." Do this a few weeks in a row, and you have a real health problem.

You need sleep to live. Your body goes through cycles of activity during sleep that you must complete to maintain and build your body and your mental processes. One of the necessary sleep activities is the REM, or rapid eye movement, cycles. You need to go through about five of these dream cycles per night. They process your day's events and collate the day's memories into the mind's memory stores.

Your brain accesses memory in the same manner that a computer accesses a data disk. The computer looks at the registry files associated with the data location, and that tells it where to look, to access the right memory. Your brain creates 'registry file' associations of new memories to similar old memories, one of the functions of the dreams that take place during the REM cycles. No cycles mean that your brain will misfile important memories. Misfiling the memories makes them hard to find. Thus, they are hard to access when you need them to help you resolve future problems.

If you have an injury, your body waits until you are sleeping to do most of the routine healing. Most of your body resources go to the waking activities and demands while you are awake. The 'down time' of sleep is the best time to heal and repair the physical and mental problems that your systems have incurred. The healing takes place when your brain predominates in producing theta and delta waves. Sleep is important to healing.

Your body also determines what to do with the excess calories that you consumed during the day. If it thinks that you are living in a hostile environment, and a future need for nutrients is more likely than a current need for energy, it will store the nutrients as fat. You will gain weight. If it thinks that you need lots of energy to be popular, make babies, and live a happy life, then it will turn all those calories into energy for you.

These body decisions take place in all three of the lowest frequency states, Alpha, Theta, and Delta. In these same states, your mind and body will work on the positive aspects of your life, which you have been trying to convince it is true. Your sleeping mind solidifies your Self-Image, and this is very important to health, weight and the components of happiness.

There is real magic in the world, and when you have strong Theta and Delta states, you are in touch with it. Your unconscious mind, which I like to call the Undermind, works to bring you anything that you tell it (in the right way) is true. If you want good things to happen, your mind creates the world view that allows it to accept these 'Truths' in a deep sleep. Then the Undermind goes to work on them, creating miraculous opportunities and amazing insights that allow you to accomplish your goals. We will cover this, in detail, in a future chapter.

Sleep is the most important need that we have, next to getting enough food, water, and shelter to survive. If we do not get enough, we suffer from infections and diseases, depression, bad memory recall, out of control weight gain, stress and an out of control life. If we go without sleep long enough, we suffer from hallucinations, mania, organ collapse, and finally death.

We have not covered the Beta state, the primary wave state of our brains while we are awake. The Beta state is a *cautious* state of mind. When we avoid possible violence, or we avoid a predator, we are thinking with the Beta state in charge. It makes us think about the world with the view that the world is a dangerous place. It is important to our species survival, but it does have one drawback. When you need to choose a 'yes' or a 'no' answer, on an 'opportunity versus risk' situation, it always says 'no.'

When deciding whether to date the person of your sexual dreams, the Beta state advises you not to risk it. If you want a 'yes,' you have to talk to the Alpha, Theta, or Delta states. That is where you will start to get some 'yeses.'

## Good Sleep:

When you get enough good sleep, those bad things that we just discussed, which the lack of sleep could bring, are just another distant nightmare. There is no downside to getting enough sleep. As for the upside, let us count the ways.

On average, in a full night's sleep, you get Five REM cycles. You sort through your day's memories and events in these. These are special active states, where the voluntary muscles are paralyzed to prevent sleepwalking, and you gain the gift of clear thoughts and memory recall from going through these cycles.

The Alpha, Theta and Delta states bracket the REM states. You get de-stressed systems, healed injuries, balanced emotions, energy and some wonderful insights and ideas for any problems you may face the next day from these obstacles. Sleep, as a whole, is the incubator for the amazing talents that you use, the successes that you enjoy, and the happiness that you find in the world. Without sleep, and pardon my French, it is all crap!

A sleeping person usually creates Good sleep by the faithful employment of good habits. You may want to take a warm bath just before bed, listen to relaxing music, and spend fifteen to thirty minutes meditating before you hit the hay. You may want to jump right into an exercise routine, an enjoyable task, or another session of meditation upon awakening. The actions that you habitually take before bed tells the body to begin preparing to sleep and the actions you habitually take after waking tells the body to start the day off right.

Some ambitious Author could write an entire book on this one part of a healthy life. In fact, many have been. If the subject interests you, there are many good books that you may want to read on the subject. For our purposes, let us just stress that sleep is vital to the issue of losing and maintaining weight. I will assume that you realize the truth of this, and we will move on to other ingredients in the buffet that we call natural weight loss.

There is one last aspect of sleep that we need to discuss. I may have mentioned earlier that this world of ours contains **real magic**. I was serious about that. Your Undermind can create amazing opportunities and to get your goals by its sheer computing power. It also connects to whatever metaphysical or spiritual parts of the universe may exist. If you believe in intuition, extrasensory perception,c or any form of magic, including the miracles of the ancient prophets, the Undermind is the part of us connected to it.

Believe it or not, your Undermind can reach out into the world around us, with powers beyond the comprehension of our waking minds, and change the world to reflect the things that we *believe*, or that we *expect* to be part of the world around us. In the context of weight loss, your Undermind can change the world, or you, in a way that causes your body to lose weight and keep it off, or any other thing that you believe, or expect.

# 7: THE SELF-IMAGE FACTOR

## Background:

**We** all carry a mental image of who we are in our minds. We will frequently take out this 'mental photograph' to look at, making sure that we know how we act and look. This image is our true face, according to our minds. We will do anything to make sure that the mental image we hold of ourselves, and our actual Self, are the same thing, even if the mental image is less than flattering.

We *are* our Self-Image. Our mental image composes the history we recall, a visualized 'snapshot' of how we think we look physically, and the beliefs about our world and ourselves that we think has a bearing on what we are. If we consider ourselves to be **unworthy** of good things, our mental image will reflect this belief, and we will filter what we recall of our histories to support this belief.

Our actions will always exactly agree with our Self-Image, even though it is only a conceptual construction. When we look in the mirror, the image that we see is not the true image of ourselves. We see our bodies filtered by the concepts that we have developed about who and what we are. Our mental pattern recognition processes always filter our senses. In this case, our minds filter out all the photonic patterns that our mental image denies existence, and it will add in mental patches of the image to make it exactly match what we *expect to see* when we look in the mirror.

Our beliefs about whom and what we are trumps any actual evidence that we might encounter of other qualities we may have. When we look in the mirror, or we consider ourselves in any way, we see only those things that we expect to see. A depressed person (such as Droopy, of cartoon fame) will see a depressed and undeserving person in the Mirror. A Narcissist (such as Donald Trump, of Political cartoon fame) will see the most wonderful person he or she knows when they look in the mirror.

Our expectations and beliefs are responsible for both our Self-Image and for how our universe treats us. If we expect to win the games, we play, for the most part, this will be so. If we expect to lose, nothing will stop us from losing. The universe will deliver an almost infinite number of events to support our beliefs, no matter what those beliefs are.

Everything that we see filters through our mental processes. Without those filters, we find ourselves submerged in a flood of stimuli well beyond our ability to see any patterns, or any order, in the world around us. We lose our minds in a world of chaos.

What we believe about the world, or about ourselves, will reach deep into the structure of our universe, and change it to conform to those beliefs. There have been many examples of this in history, and many people are credited with powers to change the world beyond any physical laws, as we understand them. Our minds can access and use these powers. True magic exists in the world, and we are either its masters or we are mastered by it.

We create new personalities for new situations all the time. When you start a new job, you will decide what you need to be to thrive in your new position, and then you will become the person that has those qualities. If you create the perfect personality fit for the job, you will move up rapidly in the company. If you make a bad fit, you will soon find yourself in the unemployment line.

We create such new Personas for our major activities. One is for our home life; one is for school, and so forth. We imagine a 'real me,' but in truth, what we think is *us* is really just the longest running Persona we created, to survive our childhoods.

If a person creates several new Personas for the same situation unconsciously and then loses control of their activations, he is said to have a mental illness known as 'Multiple Personality Disorder.' Because the person will shuffle in an uncontrolled manner between the Personas, it is not a positive condition, and the mental health officials correctly assume that he needs treatment.

One tantalizing aspect of split personalities is that each personality may exhibit very different mental and physical properties in the same body. For instance, some studies of subjects of split personalities observed that one personality might have a full-blown case of diabetes, while another personality has no diabetes condition at all! One may have a talent or skill totally lacking in another personality. One may be a whiz at science or math, with no talent for an Art, while another is an Artist with no science and math ability.

## Bad Self-Image:

When we look into the mirror, most of us see someone that could most accurately be described as either an underdog or an okay but unremarkable person. Other people and ourselves tell us that we have a limited self, most of the time, and we will usually see those limitations before we see any of the good stuff that we are.

Regarding brain waves, our opinions of ourselves are usually motivated by the Beta wave state, which will describe us by what we are not, not by what we are. When we look in the mirror, we should not look with a critical eye. When we critically observe, we are looking for deficits, not pluses. Is it any surprise that we find fault with ourselves?

Whatever the person is that we see in the mirror is our Self-Image, and we are that person, as long as we believe that we are. Our belief about ourselves, and our Self-Image, which is almost exclusively created by this belief, determines everything that we think and do in our lives. We may hide some errant fantasies about being something better, but it is what we believe we are which determines what we are.

If we believe that we are overweight, even if we are not, we will see the extra pounds on our frames when we look into the mirror. When we see ourselves as fat, we have already informed our Undermind that this is the state of affairs that we prefer. As soon as the Undermind determines that we expect this, it will start to work to make our actual body match the one we see in the mirror.

No matter what the truth, what we always expect acts as a filter on our senses, matching what we see to our expectations, and ignoring anything contrary to our expectations. As we reinforce our beliefs in our qualities, our lives, bodies and the world will conform more and more to our expectations. We will create the world we expect.

Our Undermind will reach into the fabric of the surrounding universe, and change it just enough to make the world exactly what we think it should be. If we visualize ourselves as a victim, we will become a victim. If we see ourselves as fat, we will be fat.

## Good Self-Image:

Not all is lost. You can see a better world around you, and you can see yourself as a good and worthy person, meeting the challenges of life with a slender body, and receiving the best from life. If you are calm about existence and expect only good things, the Alpha wave state is in charge, and the person in the mirror will look much more desirable than the Beta state version.

Let us take two extreme examples of the Beta state loser and the Alpha state winner. For the Beta state, let us take as our example the lamented Don Knotts. For our Alpha state, let us take as our example the bombastic Donald Trump.

Don Knotts made his career portraying a man afraid of his own shadow, expecting at any time for the universal shoe to drop, and for the sky to fall. As a consequence, the lives that he portrayed were always lives of antic failures, fun to watch, painful to live. When his characters looked into a mirror, they would always see a failure.

Don Trump is an interesting man. He is quite taken with himself. I think it is obvious that he considers himself to be better than he considers others. I cannot say that I like his personality, but it is evident he believes in himself in a big way. When he looks into a mirror, I think that he likens what he sees to the gods of old. If his mirror image had lady parts, he would probably marry it.

We all see our Self Image when we look in the mirror. We reflect our beliefs about ourselves in the glass. The mind goes to work to make sure that all perceptions we have will agree with what we expect to see. If we think that we are overweight, the mirror will add a hundred pounds. If we think that we are a slender but powerful winner, the glass will reflect that powerful winner.

Our beliefs form our expectations, and our expectations will determine our world. If the Golden Rule is the first rule of living, then the zeroth rule is that our expectations always determine our world. If you want good things to happen in your world, you must expect good things to happen. Until you absorb this fact, the bad expectations that you hold will always be in charge of your life.

Fortunately, for us, there are shortcuts that we can take to get a good life. The primary tool that we use in creating a good life is to learn how to create and properly make use of new personalities, or Personas, equipped to handle the obstacles of Life. There is nothing that is beyond your reach if the proper **You** is reaching for the prize.

We will go through the process of creating the appropriate Personas to use in a future chapter. We will devote a chapter to activating the Persona. Things will get more exciting from here!

# 8: CREATING GOALS

## Background:

**If** you want to get *any* of the things on your wish list, then you must create and work on a set of goals. Experience proves that you are *many times more likely* to get what you want out of life if you plan and write your objectives down as goals. If you work on goals, without creating the written goals, you *rarely* complete them.

Never build something without a plan is always good advice. Your life is no different. You should take the time to write down a goal, before starting to work on it. You will be creating a plan for that part of your life.

There are other reasons for writing your goals down. You have to think about the goal if you wish to write it out. Writing down your goal will flesh out the plan a lot more. You also start the process of discovering how you can do it by writing it out.

For instance, you may have a vague dream of making a million bucks. This fantasy does not supply *any* of the details that you need actually to make it happen. From where will the money come? A goal will usually make a statement. 'I will have a profit of one million dollars from my Mail Order Bride business in 2016', or some more normal statement. This will give you an area of activity to focus on, to secure the goal.

Besides being logical and physical, the statement of the goal has a more esoteric effect. Once you have formed your goal, you have begun to inform your Undermind that you actually expect this result. Your Undermind will immediately go to work to create the results it thinks you expect.

Your Undermind has a computational ability *far beyond* your conscious mind's ability to even comprehend, let alone duplicate. If any direct path to the goal exists, your Undermind *will* find it. Your Undermind also has that supernatural aspect that you have *always* known exists, which can reach out and tweak the universe around you to make it become a world within which you have that goal accomplished.

## The Procedure:

You can form your goal list by just jotting down your dreams. Have you always wanted to visit Argentina? Do you want to have a dolphin live in your swimming pool? More to the point, do you want to be at your ideal weight and in perfect health? Are you looking for that perfect sex object? You get the idea.

You should write down **everything** that you would like to be, do and have in your life. Let yourself go, and do not worry about how possible it is, or anything other than your desire for it. This might take you thirty minutes, or two hours, or several hours. After a while, you will run out of things to jot down. Congratulations, you have written down a Dream's List!

Once you have written down your dreams, take a few moments to pick out the top ten most desired dreams, and list them from most desired as number one, to least desired (of the ten) as number ten. You are going to turn these into goals to complete. Losing weight should be topping this list unless you are reading the wrong book.

Let us follow the example of the Losing weight dream, to see how to make it into a goal. Take a few moments to think about specifics, and what tools you have to make it happen. For example:

I want to lose twenty pounds and become healthier, eating the right mix of foods, exercising, and becoming a healthy, happy and more slender person, using the Chapter labeled 'The Plan' from the book 'Losing Weight Naturally as a procedural guide.

Now we need to get even more specific, adding in deadlines and then rewriting the goal as though it is in process, and we have, or almost have, completed the goal.

This will be a slightly tilted process of goal building since we are attempting to create only one or two goals which are not typical because they are compound goals, consisting of several elements, which are each sub-goals. We will be working on losing weight, increasing exercise and activity, eating a good diet, and increasing success and happiness. Each should be a goal unto itself, but since they are linked, we will treat this as one goal.

If you are looking for a more comprehensive procedure for creating and working on goals, you might like to read my book **Whacking Happiness**. I will give you the abbreviated version of the procedure in this book since it focuses on losing weight.

The next step in creating our goal is to make a deadline for some specific part of the goal so that we have something for which to shoot. Let us say that we want to lose the twenty pounds by June 1, 2016. We also need to couch the goal in terms that sound to the Undermind as though we are approaching the completion of the goal so that it thinks that we are expecting, and seeing, the results we want. Let us give it a shot now:

I will lose all twenty pounds of weight and will be at 120 pounds by June 1, 2016. I am eating a well-balanced Paleo Diet slowly and enjoying every bite each day, and every day, I pick up an additional repetition in each routine in my exercise routine. I am sleeping well, I have a wonderful social life, and every task I take on at work, and home is completed before the deadline and without problems. Every time I need something, an opportunity appears to get it. My life is better and more fun every day! I am using the chapter labeled 'The Plan' from the book 'Losing Weight Naturally as a procedural guide.

Experts in goal writing may have issues with this format, but it works pretty well for me. Notice that I specified a deadline for the primary sub-goal losing weight and couched it so that it sounds as though you are well on your way to achieving this goal, **which is true**. After all, once you decided actually to do something about your weight, aren't you **already** well down the road to losing the weight?

Think about it. Typically, this is probably the first time you have tried to do something about the problem yourself, instead of looking for a diet system, drug or counselor to solve the problem for you. Jenny Craig is probably wonderful, but do you think that you can bear to eat the canned foods, and not work to modify the rest of your habits in your life, and be successful? Me neither.

You can have a list of goals to work on, and I do not wish to discourage that. Even with simple goals, you probably should not work on more than three at a time. This goal is not simple, and it could be considered the same as several goals, so I suggest you only work on it, at least until you have achieved the primary objective of losing the weight.

At this point, I would ordinarily say that you need to rank your goals, but I suggest instead that you create those goals, write them down, and file them away for now. Your Undermind will still start working on them for you, but you want to change your life by achieving your primary goal.

The next thing you need to do is to break down the goal into a series of steps that you can complete, to reach the goal. You can focus on the exercise aspect, defining a specific exercise routine of sit-ups, push-ups, squats and such, and define a ramping up procedure for each exercise, such as adding one more repetition of each, each day.

Regarding food, you may want to dig up tasty recipes of well-balanced Paleo dishes, analyze them for proper composition and affordability, and create a weekly menu.

You certainly need to practice techniques of meditation and visualization, plan on attending social functions that give you the possibility of forming new relationships, and streamline or simplify your life to reduce distractions from your goals.

Once you have defined a series of steps that you can take to reach the goal, it is time to start working on each step in the sequence. You need to take the next step each day and jot it down on some kind of To-Do List, as a task to work on or complete today.

Fear makes most of us procrastinate. We fear larger tasks because we are not sure that we can complete them. The solution to this is in two parts. First, break down the task into manageable chunks. I write this book chapter by chapter, and only after I have taken a few moments to write out an outline of the chapter. Then, and only then, I start to write. A book may be daunting, but who cannot write a chapter?

The last part of this formula is that I immediately begin the task, once I have the tools. Do not give yourself time to get discouraged. Don't think, just do it! Once you have part of the task completed, you will be encouraged, and it will be easy!

# Lose Weight Naturally

# 9: DEFINING BELIEFS

## Background:

**Your** beliefs define *who* you are. They define your talents and your limitations. They are the part of your mental process that determines how you see the world around you. They are the **keystones** of your success or failure.

Our families give us most of our beliefs, at a young age. If somebody tells you that working hard is the only way to get ahead, you believe this. It becomes part of your core personality. It is so seldom that we change such beliefs. We usually think that we cannot change them.

The fact is that you can change your beliefs. It is easy. There are likely some examples in your own history.

Perhaps your father told you that the whole Christian worldview was true. A specific and uncontroversial set of Truths (pick your version here) is part of this belief. If you absorbed this at a young age, you might have the belief embedded in you. Later, in college, you start to doubt the spin on Christianity you learned. It doesn't seem to match up to real life. It is not that hard to align your beliefs with your new observations. You just need to be far away from the family influence.

One of the nicer aspects of your belief structure is that you must decide what you believe. When you were young, you decided to believe what your parents told you to believe. You had to choose to accept those beliefs. At any time, you may decide a belief is wrong, or that you like an alternate belief better. It is a simple choice to make the change.

We all need some beliefs to give our world meaning, and something to accomplish. You may need a belief in some god, or a higher spiritual entity. You need to believe that you occupy some position within the social structure. You need to believe that you deserve, or do not deserve, certain rewarding or punishing events. Most of us need to believe that we exist for a purpose. None of us want to believe that our existence is no more than random chance.

Whatever beliefs you have chosen, hold them as simple choices. These chosen beliefs create the expectations that you have of the world, and of yourself. Well-chosen beliefs promote expectations of good things.

Your Undermind will make any expectation you show it into a reality. This means that a chosen belief can create beneficial expectations. This instructs the Undermind to create a beneficial world for you to inhabit.

The world will always conform to your expectations.

## Bad Beliefs:

Most normal human beings absorb some bad beliefs as they grow up. Most families are not perfect, and some of the messages about what is true can be outright lies or at least fibs. One of the old and evil Communist leaders once said 'give me the children, young enough, and they are mine forever.'

It is not as bad as all that, but the younger you are, the less likely you are to reject a belief, and it becomes a core part of your personality. Self-esteem problems are hard to kick because you accepted the beliefs that created them, at a young age. They become part of who you are. The best thing to do when your personality is so flawed is to trade it in for another personality, just like you would your car.

When I was young, I was an introverted kid. I was an avid and fast reader, and I avoided people like the plague that they seemed to be. Needless to say, I was not the most assertive kid on the planet. As long as you didn't trip my stubbornness switch, you could play all sorts of bullying games with me.

One day, I got mad about the situation, and I decided to act out. It worked like a charm, as the social dynamic changed around me to accept the new behavior. After that, I experimented with asserting myself in other ways, with equal results.

Conflicting beliefs are one of the problems that you have in dealing with life. Most of us believe that it is wrong to allow anyone to force anyone else to do something they do not want to. We have also absorbed the belief that it is okay in certain situations to allow certain people to force us to do something we don't want to do. This is a conflict unless you believe that you are nobody.

The first belief is a liberating belief, and we all know that it is true. The second belief is a limiting belief, and even the believer knows that it is not objectively true. Most of us have grown up with such limiting beliefs. We just accommodate them, because we know how deep they run.

There is one problem with these limiting beliefs. They drive our expectations. If we believe that we do not deserve a good life, with all the social, financial and spiritual benefits attached to it, then we also expect that the world will deliver us a bad life, with deprivation and pain its main features.

If we lived in a wholly mechanical world, where what we expected had no great influence on what we received, this would not be that big of a problem. There is a problem. The expectations we hold, for any given outcome, are the biggest determiner of those outcomes we create.

The most common failure complexes that people have derived are of the beliefs they have that define their limitations. They grow up thinking that they cannot excel at math or science, or public speaking because they have a belief that tells them these are true.

Most limiting beliefs are bad beliefs. A few limiting beliefs have good results. One such belief is that one cannot fly when perched on the side of a cliff. Many limiting beliefs act to keep us within our comfort zones. This can be okay, provided we are happy there.

Here is a summary of bad beliefs. Bad beliefs are beliefs which cause us not to do and be those things that we would desire to be. Bad beliefs are based on our acceptance of limitations, and they create bad expectations for our future and present world. This causes unresolved stress and the other unhealthy effects in our bodies. It tells our Undermind that we expect the bad world that we have visualized.

Our Undermind starts to work immediately, creating the world that our expectations have been telling it that we wanted. The Undermind has no concern with the sort of world it creates for us. It is equally happy with a life of torture and death, as it is with a life that is heaven on earth. It just does what we tell it, and how we tell it is by expecting the world to be a certain way.

## Good Beliefs:

A few of us were lucky to have grown up with mostly good beliefs imposed upon us. The world that this made for us supports the creation of even more good beliefs. We enjoy the fruits of good expectations.

Most of us were not lucky enough to be born into such a well-adjusted family. Most of us inherited a few good beliefs and a mountain of bad beliefs. It is lucky for us that we can change the mix of beliefs we have. It can be a simple process, and then we can have the lives we want to live.

Consider the belief in God. We have a choice of believing in God, or not to believe. It is a simple choice, as long as we do not see evidence that points the other way, or as long as we do not accept that evidence.

A good example is a belief in UFOs. There is insufficient evidence to prove the UFO activity is actually due to alien incursions into our skies. Most of the Contactees reporting the events insist that it is aliens. Most examples of reported UFOs we find to be commonplace events, such as airplane or helicopter flights, or weather events. There are still thousands that seem to be non-normal events.

There is little doubt that something is happening, and that is the definition of an unidentified flying object. There is no doubt about the existence of this reality, but many confronted with this evidence can still believe that UFOs are not real, and some will insist that UFOs are real, without even considering the evidence.

We do choose our beliefs. We even choose our long-held beliefs. It just takes a little more reweaving of our personalities, or a personality makeover in the form of a new created Persona.

We have to decide what beliefs will benefit us to have unless we want our world determined by random chance, and people are imposing beliefs upon us who were not considering our benefit when they defined our worlds for us.

What we must do to change our world is simple. First, we must determine what beliefs would be of benefit to us in having the world we desire. Second, we must pick up a pen and paper, and write the beliefs down. Third, we must imagine ourselves living in the world where these beliefs determine our worlds.

The imagining process is by the use of daydreaming, meditation, visualization and by working on the goals that we have in the real world. This will reinforce the expectations that we pass along to our Undermind, and cause the beliefs, the goals, and the world to become real.

# 10: DESCRIBE YOUR PERSONA

## Background:

**We** *are* our Personas. The person that you see staring back at you out of the mirror is not a simple reflection of photons. Your mind takes the light it sees in your reflection. It adds everything that it believes that you are, into the image that the brain receives.

From the time that you were in your mother's womb, you have received information from the world. This told you things about whom and what you were. Some of these earliest ones were hormonal injections into your body. These may have produced emotional states such as depression or a feeling of security. All these things, you added into your self-image.

As soon as you were born, you began to hear comments about you that you had to consider true. Some of these were good comments, producing good personality traits. Most of them were bad. Beliefs, about whom and what you are, were born in those minutes.

You started to expect the world to treat you a certain way as you grew. These expectations depended on what qualities you believed the world, and yourself possessed. As soon as you expected a specific outcome of events, your Undermind would go to work to deliver it to you. This reinforced your beliefs and your expectations. It was a massive feedback loop.

Each time you looked into the mirror, you would note that what you saw was a more advanced version of what you expected to see. You see what you expect in the mirror. If you think you are fat, you see yourself as fat. The question is, how do you change what you see?

Consider what an actor would do. When you were in grade school, I am sure that you were in a play or two, and you found it hard to portray the character you were playing. You worked hard to deliver the lines, but it always felt a little stilted. You didn't put the emphasis on your lines where it belonged, and your verbal and physical actions were not well timed. What is different about how a good actor goes about acting as the character?

Give a veteran actor a script to read, and he will come back to you with questions. What is the character's motivation? What is the character's history? What does he look like when the character looks in the mirror? After many such questions, the Actor will create a mental history of the character. This will explain the identity of the character.

Soon, the Actor has a firm grasp on the character's history, his beliefs, and how he appears. He is now ready to portray him. When he starts reciting the lines, the Actor has become the character he is playing. He has played scenarios of the character, and his actions, in his mind many times, and he *is* the character.

What the Actor has done is to create a Persona, based upon the character he must play. It is simple for him to put the Persona on, and react to life and situations as the Character. Actors are good at this, but we all can do the same thing. In fact, we all have done this many times in our lives. It is a subconscious process that we use to fit into new situations. We need to create our new Persona consciously like the Actor does. If we do that, we can control what we will become while wearing it.

### Bad Persona:

Most of us have major problems. The Personas that we have created for ourselves reflects these problems. If we have problems accepting Authority, this sometimes is incorporated into our Work Persona. It is sure to make trouble with our Boss.

Our Self-Esteem is a pervasive aspect of our core personality. We usually incorporate it into our situational Personas. If you have bad self-esteem issues, they will usually crop up in any Persona you create. This is because you instinctively created your new Persona, using the old personality as the base format. You only changed the bits of yourself that needed to be changed to do the specific job.

This means that your new Persona usually will have the *same problems* that your original personality does. This is an easy fix, if you build the new Persona carefully, and expect it to be an improvement on, and replacement for, the original personality.

The person looking out at you from the mirror is flawed. What do you expect, when that personality has grown like a weed, in poor soil, and with little or no tending? Imagine what a godlike Persona you could create to wear, if you did a little *planning*!

You maintain your old beliefs, your old history, and change your personality only slightly to create the new **You**. Why would you expect the world to treat the new **You** better than it did the old **You**?

This is the reason that the new employee gets into trouble with his boss. It is why the new student has a problem with the college life. It is why most new business owners cannot make a go of their new business.

We all have seen the incompetent employee that keeps failing upwards. We sat next to the student who is awful at learning, that keeps getting A grades. We know the business owner who is downright stupid, but who still runs a thriving business. Guess what they have, that you lack? In a miraculous session of thought, using their one good neuron, they managed to make a Persona that expected to succeed in what they were doing.

If such train-wrecks as these can make a go of it, by the creation of a proper personality, or Persona, to do the job, imagine what you can do. The only true limitations you have are the ones you put on yourself. You can be slender, healthy, creative, and productive faster than you ever thought was possible.

71

## Good Persona:

Think about the stupid business owner. He has an IQ of 80, a one-dimensional personality, and an expectation of the ability to run and expand his company. If he were to depend solely on his abilities, he would have to pack it in. **Something** exists which is more important.

We are all inherently competent to do almost anything that we can conceive. Even our poor brain damaged business owner has all the tools he needs to do whatever he wants. The fact that we have more tools than he does just does not matter. He believes, and we do not.

The bottleneck of our success **is not** our abilities. We all have plenty of those. The only true obstacle is our belief in ourselves, our abilities, and what the world will let us get, and keep.

Let us reference religion here. The Bible says that if you have even the smallest faith (the size of a mustard seed), you can move mountains. You can ask from the world whatever you would, and the world will deliver it to you. What the Bible calls faith, we call Belief.

If you believe in God, and that he will answer your prayer, then you expect an appropriate result when you pray for success in whatever activity you are engaged. Faith in God creates Belief that you will have desired outcomes of events. The Belief stimulates your Undermind to create the expected result. Everyone goes home happy.

Think about it. A Kennedy grows up expecting a wonderful life, where he gets anything he wants. He is seldom wrong. The fortunate lad who grows up in a loving and supportive family gets good grades easily, a full ride to a great college, and a lucrative position at a major employer, with all the perks. These are his expectations, and he is not disappointed.

Isn't it time that you got some of the good life? It is a simple recipe to cook up some Successful **You**. There are only three ingredients. One part each history, beliefs, and self-image, mix well and enjoy.

If you have not already completed these tasks, you need to imagine the perfect you, describe yourself, what you believe, what your history is, and what you will do in the future.

## Creation:

Describe to yourself how you look. What is important to you, and what talents and activities you are a genius at using and doing? Write out at least one page that describes how your new Persona looks. What makes him the Ideal you?

The next page will describe the beliefs that your new Persona holds. At the bottom, maybe a few scribbles about what negative beliefs you have, that you do not want the new You to have would be valuable.

Imagine the new **You**, and end each one of your daily meditations (you are doing that, right?) with a visualization of the new **You**. End the visualization by getting up and looking into the mirror. Force the new **You** that you visualized to be the image you see in the mirror.

I know that this all seems a little simplistic, but it will work if you do it. Keep at it, follow the rest of the book instructions, and you will lose the weight. You will feel better about yourself. You will start to get things that you never thought that you would have, do, or become.

# 11: MEDITATION AND VISUALIZATION

## Background:

**We** all visualize our world and ourselves every day. Our visualizations consist of fantasy actions and conversations and daydreaming. They also consist of mental images of events, ourselves and all parts of the world around us. We can visualize anything we wish to visualize, with a little training.

Visualization is a mental process, where we stimulate our optic nerves. We mentally produce a picture or an image of something. Our brains and minds are not able to differentiate a visualization from 'the reality' of actually seeing the event. This comes in quite handy when trying to convince your Undermind that what you want to happen has a history of happening, and so, you expect it to happen again.

When we visualize some part of our world, it is the first step in manifesting that quality or event in our world. When we visualize ourselves, we are visualizing our self-image. If we want to change our self-image, we need to visualize a more *desirable* version of our self.

Our Undermind is a machine that blindly seeks to give us what it sees that we expect. If we want to change ourselves, the simple way to do this is to change our expectations. Whatever we believe, we generate expectations based on those beliefs. Whatever we expect, our Undermind will make real for us.

## Bad Visualization:

In a very real sense, we generate our viewpoint of our world within a dream from which we never wake. If you think about the quality of consciousness, you find that, at its core, the same dream quality exists that defines you as the dreamer within your nightly dreams.

All of our fears and our needs constantly murmur in the back of our minds. Our decisions are made subconsciously to avoid certain situations and to seek out others. We have a mental image of what the world is like, just as sharp and potent to our actions as is the mental image we hold of who we are.

For most people, the big problem is that we have a strong belief that the universe will dish out bad stuff to us soon. Because we are thinking about the possible future events while we are awake, the primary mental frequency involved is the Beta wave state of brain activity.

When Beta waves are primary, we tend to be ultra-cautious. We are too ready to fall into the 'fight or flight' mode of action. This predisposes us to believe that future events will be bad for us. With practice, we can learn to live our waking lives mostly in an Alpha state, calm and relaxed, and promoting generally positive attitudes toward future events.

Your mind works very much like a genie. Rub the lamp, and the genie comes out to grant you whatever wish you want granted. The Rubbee never seems to have a handle on phrasing his wishes right, and they always end in disaster. Do any of the lucky recipients of a genie ever get good things from their wishes?

In the Beta state, we tend to ask for things of the universe that we do not want or need that much. We ask for a million bucks when all we really want is to enjoy the next year in peace. If you think about it, we tend to ask for the resources to protect ourselves from a hostile universe, when we are in Beta.

Bringing the subject back to the main focus of this book, in the Beta state, we might ask to lose twenty pounds. In the Alpha state, we might ask to be healthy and happy. In the Beta state, losing the pounds is very hard. In the Alpha state, it is a consequence of our happy pursuit of our goal, and we may not even notice as the pounds melt away.

## Good Visualization:

A fortunate few of us have a good self-image and a good perspective on the world around us. Usually, this is a result of growing up in a sane and nurturing family, supported in achieving our goals, and living in an environment that **encourages** us to try new things and enjoy living.

If the last paragraph doesn't describe you, do not despair. Plants can be lucky to sprout in good conditions, but you can also plant and tend them, and you wind up with another healthy plant. It does not mean that you are lost just because your childhood was not perfect. We can create, intentionally, the life you should have had.

The procedure for getting your life, and all of its parts, on the right path, is simple. Decide what you want. Write down your goals. Choose Beliefs that benefit you. Decide who you would like to be. Create that new Persona, and become it. Expect the same things you desire. Start working on your goals.

Put in a concerted effort to do these things, and I guarantee you will improve your life by thousands of percentage points. Do them correctly, and you will be healthy, happy, and will not suffer from self-esteem related problems, such as weight problems.

It is not that hard to imagine a good life. We all have a generic idea of what a good life would be like, floating around in our heads. It probably features plenty of money, free time, loving relationships, health, and interesting events. It is a collection of generalities, a blurry, unfocused vision of what the world would be like if we had 'the good life.'

The biggest problem that most people have is not making plans. If you go vacationing, you know where you want to go, and you map out the route to get there. If we applied the same amount of planning to our lives that we do to vacations, we would be most of the way to having that wonderful life we seek.

Once we have decided to plan our life, by creating goals and changing our habits, beliefs, and Persona, we have to check our tools and complete the job. We check our goals, beliefs, and habits for value to us. We start to work our goals. By the way, the way you know that you are correctly working goals is that you get lost in them. You parcel out a half hour to do part of a goal step and discover that the next time you come up for air, it has been eight hours, you got a lot done, and you enjoyed every second of it.

If we imagine a good life, plan it out, write it down, and start to work the steps, we can expect good things. Our conscious minds are like your pet crocodile. It is hard to train the crocodile not to look at the Feeder as food, but it will slowly realize that not eating the Feeder benefits it more than one big meal. Our Beta mind is pessimistic, but with enough evidence of progress, even without the most exotic changes that I am advocating here, it will still start to get more optimistic, and even start expecting good things.

Once you start expecting the good life, whether you achieve that end by the easy or the hard route, your Undermind will start working to create that life for you.

## Visualization:

We are always living in a daydream. Our conscious processes are composed of two primary parts. Our identity is a recursive feedback loop, where every event we encounter we refer to our self-image that we carry around, acting as a filter of data to make it relevant to our existence. If we were a computer, instead of wetware, we would see our conscious identity as a complicated If-Then subroutine. By the time a piece of data has made it through this recursive subroutine, we can now fit it into our data files in the way most conducive to the continuation of our identity.

Our minds very heavily edit our sensory inputs. To use and retain any specific information, we have to attach meaning to it, and we have to associate it with other data that we have already stored away. This is the reason that strange experiences, such as alien contact, supernatural experiences, and even picnics with Bigfoot, are so hard to process. They do not fit with our more mundane experiences.

Dreams are all about meaning. Every action in a dream is chock full of meaning. The only way you realize that you are dreaming is that things happen there that you know does not happen in 'real life.' The weird thing is that 'real life' is actually a special dream state. We think of our minds as composed of several different mind states. We think that we are awake, or asleep, experiencing the real world, or a dream world. Conventionally, we even think that the Beta, Alpha, Theta, and Delta states are distinct and separate. Neither of these assumptions is true.

Our identity feedback loop makes 'real life' seem egocentric. Our base experience is a dream state with identity and 'real life' problems and events featured prominently. Our Beta state adds a touch of fear and nightmare to the mix. Our deep Undermind sees what we experience, and it assumes that whatever we experience is what we want, so it treats the unplanned life events as a reorder situation. Whatever happened to us yesterday, it assumes we want more of the same tomorrow.

In a very real sense, we are trapped in a dream. It can be a bad scene, or it can be wonderful. The Undermind brings you the life you expect, so why not change what you expect into what you want. If you can visualize a better life, your Undermind cannot tell that it did not happen, so it will try to give you more of the same. Let us cover a short introduction to visualization.

If you figure out a specific change to your life that you would like to make, imagine for a moment a scene, just like in a movie, where you see yourself getting that change. Let me tell you what I would do next.

I close my eyes, and imagine myself in my Mind Palace, sitting in a darkened room at its center. Energy is discharging everywhere around me, like static discharges to the level of lightning voltages, but when they touch me, I only feel the energy, and a general healing as they pass through me.

I watch this for a while, while the energy heals me, and calms me, and takes me deep through the Alpha state, into the Theta state. When I feel like it, I start a movie in my mind. On this movie screen, I watch as the positive events that I imagined plays out on the screen in front of me. If I feel like it, I may run the movie several times. When I finally roll the end credits, I return to the sensation of the energy field, and mentally 'dismiss' the process.

This is a very simple method of visualization, and the initial visuals can be very effective in creating a meditative state. Do this every day, and slowly, but surely, your life will get better, and your problems will start to recede.

# 12: METAPHYSICS

## Background:

**The** Bible states that it takes only the faith the size of a mustard seed to cause a miracle to happen. It is only necessary to believe that something can happen, to *make* it happen. I would restate this to say that all, which is necessary to *change* the world we live in, is to *expect* it.

In Quantum Mechanics, events are unresolved without an Observer. If five possible outcomes exist for an event, without an Observer, all five of these outcomes are equally real, or unreal. Only when an Observer is present, will one of these outcomes resolve itself. It becomes the real one, and the other four becomes unreal.

This traditional view of Quantum Mechanics does not posit the Many Worlds Theory. The Many Worlds Theory says that the other four outcomes are ***equally real***. They branch off into parallel universes, being the real outcome in their respective universe. According to this view, the Observer only makes the fifth outcome real for ***his*** universe.

No matter which variation of Quantum Mechanics you accept, the importance of the Observer implies that Mind is integral to the definition of reality. I believe there is overwhelming evidence for the validity of the Many Worlds interpretation of Quantum Mechanics. In each interpretation, the Mind is a key component.

The standard theory would have you believe in some esoteric quality to the presence of the Observer. The presence of the Observer collapses the probabilities to permit only one reality from manifesting. The demonstrated effects of the existence of all the probabilities upon the world around us are either ignored or pointed to, as the debate requires.

One key characteristic of the universe seems to escape their notice. The expectations of the Observer, concerning an event, are rarely disappointed. Consciousness is a thing of dispute. The viewpoint of that entity with possible consciousness is entirely understandable.

There is an experiment where the Observer is absent during the emission of a single photon (particle of light). The experiment aims the photon at a series of slits in front of a photographic plate. When the Observer is present, the light acts as a particle, going through only one of the available slits. When he is not present, the light goes through all the slits, as demonstrated by the interference pattern on the exposed plate.

We usually assume that the difference is the consciousness of the observer. It is of interest that the Observer will usually expect light to act as a particle, and in his presence, the light behaves that way. Doesn't that tell you that the expectations of the Observer are important to the resolution of the quantum state?

You own a powerful engine of change, in the form of your mind. It causes your expectations to manifest in the world. It works in complex ways to manipulate events and opportunities in your world. It uses calculation and creative thought processes in the normal way. It also reaches into the fabric of reality. It changes your world on the quantum level to meet your expectations of the world.

This is why the world around you seems **supernaturally** able to dish out more of what you expect. This is regardless of the damage or benefit to you. Your Undermind will do this work every day of your life. It is your job to tame the beast. You must make it do what you want it to do.

## Bad Expectations:

A few of us expect only good things of life. For the most part, they get what they expect. Most of us expect life to dish out both good and bad events, and we get that as well. Some persons expect life to give them only bad events, and they get this as well.

You have met the unlucky ones. They expect only bad things to happen to them. They suffer depression, and they give up early in any activity important to them. They may go to hundreds of job interviews, always with rejections. They are the world's worst salesmen. Casinos depend on them to make the casino rich.

They get exactly what they expect out of life. Their childhoods condition them, along with past events, to expect to fail at everything they do. Even in the rare event where they get a good result, their mind will ignore or forget the one good jewel in the middle of the cesspool that has become their life.

Their Undermind is busy, getting them everything they expect. They find ample evidence in every day to prove to them that they are failures in life. They have created a feedback loop that strengthens their belief in their failure hood. This then strengthens their expectations of failure. This in turn causes the Undermind to work even harder to make them the failure they expect to be.

The characteristic most affecting this group is that what they expect is completely different from what they want in life. They want money, and relationships, and all the other good things that everyone wants. They do not expect any of those things to work out well for them.

## Good Expectations:

The few with only good expectations of life receive what they expect as well. They can look into their past and find a great deal of evidence that they are the winners they expect to be.

They go to a small number of job interviews. Then the biggest problem they have is to decide which wonderful position they want.

They find a boyfriend or girlfriend when they want one, and they marry the person they want. When they have families, it is a good, functional family. Money almost *magically* appears in their bank accounts. They get vacations, houses, and automobiles whenever they want them. They are as blessed as the Losers are cursed.

The characteristic that is most in effect with this group is that what they expect is the same as what they want in life. They want money, and relationships, and all the other good things that everyone wants, and they expect all those things to work out well for them. Because they want and expect the same things, their Undermind works hard to bring them exactly what they want.

Each experience they had worked to reinforce their expectation of good outcomes for all the events in their lives. They are the living incarnation of a well-known rule of life. They who have gets.

## The Rest of Us:

Most of us have mixed expectations. We expect to get a few good things and have a couple of bad things. Our Aunt Ethel dies (bad), but she leaves us an inheritance (good). Our lives become a mosaic of white tiles (good outcomes) with a smattering of black tiles (bad outcomes) just to keep us awake.

We only want the good things, some of our expectations match our desires, and some of them do not. This is why we get a mixed bag of luck in life.

# 13: DIET AND ACTIVITY

## Background:

**To** drop your body to its proper weight, you must eat the *right* way. This consists of eating the right things, in the right way, at the right times. You must always realize when you are eating, that the plenty available to you is unnatural. We evolved to find food in a landscape of famine. You must create a proper plan of action for eating. If you eat when you are not starving, you are doing it wrong.

For the last hundred years, the American people, and to a lesser extent the rest of the world, have had a surplus of food available to them. They ate when they wanted to, and they were dismayed when they became overweight. This led to a completely new market in the area of weight loss.

Many enterprising entrepreneurs have begun to market various diets, and diet products, in a big way. They pry the dollars from our increasingly rotund population. I am not one to object to a money loving approach to weight loss. I do object to products that increase the problems, rather than solving them.

Many approaches to dieting have appeared over the last few decades. They have usually been of either a 'balanced' or an 'unbalanced' menu. The 'balanced diets' usually use the high grain, low protein, and high dairy FDA food pyramid as a basis.

The unbalanced diets are the familiar lopsided base that we know. One Diet may suggest that we eat a low carbohydrate menu. Another suggests a high carbohydrate menu. One suggests low protein, while another suggests high protein. In each case, you must eat one category of food while avoiding every other category. I expect any day now to see an 'eat only candy' diet.

The problem with the balanced menu is that the authorities do not seem to have any true concept of what humans should eat. We are omnivores. While we can eat almost anything in a pinch, we cannot live in good health with a high grain, low protein diet. We are not designed to be Vegetarians. We are not horses.

The problem with all these diets is that the 'experts' have a poor understanding of what a human is. They do not understand that cholesterol is a normal and beneficial substance in the human body. Its presence in high concentrations in the body is an indicator of a need for body healing and repair. It is not the cause of the problem.

They do not understand that the human body was designed to forage for food in a landscape of famine. Our bodies are good at selecting and using the proper foods under famine circumstances. The foods that our unconditioned minds seek out to eat are very nutritionally rich foods. They are suitable for keeping a starving person alive.

The same foods, which cause health issues when consumed in too large quantities, are nearly perfect foods for the starving person. Eggs are a prime example of this. An egg will keep a person alive for quite some time. If they do not need the power supplied by the egg to continue surviving, the body will store it as fat instead.

The healthiest diet of a human is one where he is on the edge of a starvation diet. He is getting enough of each needed nutrient to keep the body going, but supplying nothing extra to store as fat. The person, under these conditions, reaps many mental and physical benefits. One of these benefits is a substantially enhanced life span.

Our genetics evolved to survive in a mineral rich environment. Our genes began as sea life, during a time when the mineral content of the underwater environment was less than today. It was still much higher than current soil contents. Over the eons, rain runoff has transported minerals in our soil into the seas. This left the soil mineral-poor, and the oceans increasingly mineral rich.

Having mineral-poor soil means that the food grown in that soil is also mineral poor. Our bodies recognize the lack and will attempt to make up for the deficiency, by overeating. Poor understanding of soil chemistry has allowed modern techniques in various areas to contribute to the loss of nutritional minerals.

The modern 'experts also misunderstand our metabolic system.' They assume that having all of the needed substances available means that it is a good food choice. They equate the presence of all the amino acids composing proteins to mean that these component amino acids cover the protein nutrition needs. They are wrong. There are many precursors for needed compounds in the body that the body will not be able to use, in building the compound needed. It has a set cookbook of processes to get value out of certain substances. Other substances with all the same ingredients will not work. Thinking that it will work is like thinking that crude oil is good food. All those long string hydrocarbons have everything a body needs to grow, right?

This is the common mistake that exists in the Vegan diet. They believe that a mixture of nonmeat foods will supply the body with all the proteins it needs. It would probably work for a cow, but humans are omnivores, and omnivores get their protein from animal sources. Various other deficiencies in the Vegan diet lead to nutritional deprivation. This then leads to damage to body organs, brain damage, and psychological issues.

Your sense of smell, coupled with your hunger stimuli system is among the best systems to seek out, and get, needed substances ever to exist. A prime example is the strange cravings that most pregnant women experience during their term. They will demand the most unusual foods that you can imagine. This is their body seeking out and ingesting nutritional components that the baby needs to form.

## Bad Diets:

The typical American over-eats. He is not active. He is isolated from most situations that would promote healthy activity and interactions. Many of them consider themselves overweight. The doctors agree.

There are many reasons for the problem of unhealthy weight. Humans are goal-oriented animals, and most humans never develop usable goals. Humanity is now drowning in a huge flood of foods. He overuses antibiotics and other chemicals, destroying the balance of intestinal flora. This causes the metabolic system to store fat and compromises the immune system. The foods that are available are not well balanced with vitamins, minerals and other trace compounds that we need in our diets. This causes overeating to secure an adequate amount of these substances.

Our foods are deficient in needed nutrients for many reasons. The mineral-poor soil is used to raise plants, which are also mineral poor. We eat those plants, and our bodies are not nourished by what we eat. We keep eating to supply the lacking minerals. We frugally pack the excess calories away as fat, even as we starve for the missing minerals.

Our modern world usually fertilizes our croplands with fertilizer which supplies replacement nitrogen and calcium. Modern fertilizer *does not replace* the other fifty or more needed minerals. In olden times, the fertilizer would have been waste organic materials. They would have included human and animal fecal material, garbage, and even animal organs not consumed. We do not use them as fertilizer now. We suffer from the choices we make.

Regardless of why we eat an unbalanced diet, the sum effect is that we will compulsively overeat. Huge quantities of empty calories from eating grain, and starches and sugars, are stored in the body as fat. Besides making us fat, this eating process also promotes a more lethargic lifestyle than is healthy for us.

If you have ever watched a cat, you will be aware of how they live. Give them all the food they want, and they will take a long nap right after gorging on the food. Once they wake up, they have an overwhelming urge to leap about and practice their stalking skills. If we were as wise as cats, we would also play ferociously after any bout of overeating.

One of the behaviors we share in common with the other animals is our tendency to eat as fast as we can. In the wild, this speed eating would ensure that we got the required amount of food into our system before a tiger came to chase us away from the food. In the modern world, speed eating just ensures that we overeat before our hunger stimuli can adjust to our intake, and tell us we are full.

Fad diets are poor nutrition and empty calories by their very nature. Almost all of them are extremely lopsided (nutritionally speaking), and people that use them tend to cheat on the diet one way or another. Even the ones that attempt to be balanced get it wrong. Take Jenny Craig menus. They tend to be too low in fats, too high in refined sugars, and the portions are excessively small for anyone to be satisfied with them. You are better off just nibbling on a piece of celery in the corner.

Attempting to use commercially available diet plans to lose weight will cause the average person to gain weight. The only plus to following these plans are that they do increase your exercising in one way. After becoming discouraged enough, you will doubtlessly be found on the couch doing multiple beer curls while watching television.

## Good Diet:

There are things you can do to help you stay slender, healthy, and active. It does not take much to change your eating habits radically, and ultimately your diet.

Let us consider first things first. When you have a meal, you should dish out a relatively small portion, and chew it very slowly. It is much better to have several extremely small meals during the day than it is to have one, two, or three meals. You also should be active between meals. The last meal of the day should be the smallest one. This is the one traditionally called supper, the meal where you would 'sup' just enough for you to sleep, without being distracted by hunger.

No matter how little you have eaten, when you are dining, you should stop as soon as you are satiated. In this context, read satiated as 'not hungry.' Your meals should consist of a good balance of meats, fruits, nuts, and vegetables, along with a relatively small portion of grains. If you are of European or some other dairy tolerant descent, you can wash the meal down with a glass of milk.

In ancient times, fires were frequent and rarely fought by humans. The fire turned the waste plant matter into ashes and killed off most of the parasitic types of insects. The ashes that derived from dead trees were laden with all those wonderful trace minerals that the topsoil lacked, due to the deep root system of the trees. The ashes from forest fires and chimney sweepings supplied minerals that wound up in the vegetables raised. When possible, eating foods with ashes supplementing the fertilizer would be a good addition to your menu.

Your diet should consist of some version of the Paleo Diet. This diet attempts to discover what foods have been eaten the longest by your ancestors and then duplicating that diet. The assumption is that the longer your relatives have eaten that food, the better you will be at processing it, and the less likely it is to be a cause of allergic reactions.

There are websites all over the internet that will supply you with an endless source of good Paleo recipes. Use Google to find some of them, and I will start you off with this one:

http://paleoleap.com/

One final problem with our modern diet is the presence of genetically modified plants that may be causing any number of problems with our nutritional processes. Among the most modified foods are corn and soybeans. I would avoid most soybean products, due to hormonal interruptions caused by ingesting them. The corn modification is mostly known to make the corn more pesticide tolerant, and may even be producing their own pesticides. That is probably not healthy, regardless of why pesticides saturate the grain.

You are eating most optimally if you are slightly hungry most of the time, without experiencing weakness due to starvation. After your system acclimatizes, you will find that many of your talents are enhanced, and you will age measurably slower.

When it comes to exercise, remember the cat. Eat well, get plenty of sleep, and then go play your little brains out!

# 14: YOUR NEW PERSONA

## Background:

I have a surprise for you. You are wearing a Persona right now. You may be alone. In that case, the Persona you wear is what you think of as your core personality. It will still have all the parts and mechanisms of a true Persona.

As I have stated before, a Persona is composed of three parts. It has a set of beliefs, about itself and the world around it. It has a description of itself that acts as a mental image to which it refers in all visually based thought processes. It has a history, which it can refer to for reinforcing the expectations of events, and the beliefs it holds.

A person will succeed or fail, in the ventures that they engage in depending on how well, or how badly, the beliefs and the expectations they have work to produce the events desired. You may desire a rich life of pursuing and obtaining your dreams. Unless the beliefs held by your current Persona causes you to expect to realize those dreams, you will be disappointed.

We all wear many Personas in our lives. As we are growing up, we develop one to deal with our daily life at home. We continue to mutate that Persona to deal with our daily life as we grow. We think of it as our personality, and we think that it is US. It is deep-rooted, but it is no more what we are than any of the other Personas we create over time.

We develop our School Persona as soon as we hit grade school or even Kindergarten. It exists to deal with an environment different from our home life. This Persona will continue to change, to incorporate new elements of school life, as we advance through the grades.

Some time in our early life, our social interactions become an important part of our lives. Dating, friendships, and networking are activities that need a social personality. We develop our social Persona to deal with the odd stresses of the new arena.

While we are going to college, wearing our new social Persona when not in class, we party a little too much, and so the college invites us to move back in with our family. Mother will have none of that, and father gives us a choice. We can get a job and move out, or we can move out and live under a local bridge.

We decide to play a sneaky move, so we go down to our local Army Recruiters. A couple of days later, we are shipped off to Boot Camp, with a crew cut and an urgent need for a Military Persona. Thanks to a drill Sergeant, we develop one at record speed.

For a long time, everyone else is in charge of us. We finally part ways with the uniformed life. We use our dwindling funds to rent an apartment and look for a job that will pay better than a minimum wage. We quickly develop a Job Hunting Persona, to cope with those wonderful interview questions.

One of our interviews finally pays off. They reluctantly decide to hire us. We now have to fit in. We mutate our current wardrobe of Personas, to make one that can deal well with the workplace.

Worldly success breeds worldly interest from the available prospective mates. One of them tricks us into spending money on her or him and makes us think it is a good deal. This necessitates a mutation of the old Social Persona, plus a little mental illness. She or he talks you into cohabitation with a contract. This is also known as marriage.

Marriage requires a constantly mutating Persona, as you go from the dating to fiancé, to house Frau or Hubby. Then the spawn changes things as they emerge, like the aliens from the movie 'Alien.' There are times when you suspect that marriage is God's little punishment. You continue to change, to make it work.

The point is that we all create many Personas over our lives. How well they fit the need determines how successful we are in life. If we want to get those things we desire in life, we need a well-constructed Persona.

We create most of our Personas unconsciously, and with minimal changes to the core Persona, just enough to handle the new situation. Some Personas carry over an unconscious belief that we should fail, and so they serve to close doors for us. Some are not well constructed, and so they produce poor results. If we consciously create the new Persona, we can aim it more accurately at the task it needs to complete.

A well-constructed Persona is capable of overcoming almost any obstacle. Why in the world would you leave it to chance? We have covered what a Persona is in former chapters. We have established the need for a new one to work the magic in our lives that will shed the pounds. It should also shed the other forms of self-restraint that we have been using to restrain ourselves.

You have been urged to describe your new Persona in previous chapters. Much of this chapter should be simple repetition for you. Even so, we will go through the procedure for creating and activating a Persona in this chapter.

### Bad Persona:

We all know the unlucky guy who never gets anything he wants. The universe stacks the laws of chance against him. His intelligence, skills, appearance, and any other quality he may have need not be lacking in any way for him to be the unlucky person he is.

All that it takes to be this unlucky fellow is to lack goals or to have negative goals created by negative expectations of life. He will have negative beliefs, where he is unworthy. He may in some other way feel he is deserving of bad results.

The bad expectations of Mr. Unlucky will create bad experiences for him. These will all become part of the validating history. His mind will point to this as what he is. The expectations of bad results will be strengthened for future events. Bad expectations create bad events. This creates a feedback loop reinforcing the negative expectations. Around and around he goes. The only possible final destination for him is a gutter.

Mr. Unlucky has created new Personas to deal with the new situation. The bad expectations of his core Persona carried over into each new Persona. This will bring him bad results in any situation in which he finds himself.

## Good Persona:

Other people are like Mr. Lucky. Every task he sets himself is a success. When he went to college, his grades were As, he got the girl, and he probably was the quarterback on the college team. Mr. Lucky's secret is that he has some positive goals that he enjoys pursuing. He is lucky to have inherited positive beliefs about the world and himself that serve him well. They give him good expectations about the future.

He has many successes. Each one becomes a part of his personal history. This sucessful personal history feeds his expectations of future successes and is a positive feedback loop. This strengthens his beliefs, promoting his goals, and solidifying his expectations. He is a lucky devil!

Mr. Lucky has created new Personas to deal with new situations just like Mr. Unlucky did. The positive expectations of his core Persona carried over into the new Personas, and he did well in any situation in which he found himself.

## Activation:

Now it is time to create the New Persona, and activate it. I expect you to have written out a few goals by now, one of which will be to lose the pounds that you wish to lose. You also should have sorted through your beliefs, and added some good ones to help you to reach your goals. You will have identified the bad beliefs that you hold. You have denied them a place in your belief structure.

You should already have described your new Persona to yourself. You know how you look wearing it. You know how you think, and act, while wearing it. You know that it is *you* just as much as the bad Persona that you wore when you got into your problems. It is time to change.

1. Take a moment to restate your top three goals, and write them down again. Since this is a book about losing weight, I expect the first goal will be to lose the unwanted pounds.

Once you have written all three goals down, it is time to take goals #2 and #3 and tuck them away. Every day, you should take them out and read them, but you will not be consciously working on them for a while.

2. Take out your list of beliefs that you have constructed. Think about how each one can help you lose the weight you wish to lose, put them in order of value to losing that weight, and write them down in that order. Now, memorize them in that order. As you memorize them, visualize yourself believing them in a pure and straightforward way.

3. Take out your description of the new Persona. If you have left any details out of the description, add them in now. Make sure that you know exactly how the Persona will look when you look in the mirror. I will give you a hint. It will be a thinner, healthier, nicer, and nobler version of you than any version you have previously seen or imagined. If your description does not weigh less than your normal personality did, do it again until you get it right.

4. Close your eyes and imagine the new **You**, walking and talking and feeling good. Spend lots of time in a fantasy construction of just what it will be like to be that person. You will do this every day until you are that person in *every* detail.

5. It is now time to run the Movie that you have previously created (mentally) of the Persona in action. If you have not constructed a mental movie yet, take a moment and make it now. It should center around a simple action that you (as your Persona) will take, and you will see your slender and healthy self moving as you complete the action. The following items will be the process whereby you will run that movie.

6. Set down in a comfortable position and close your eyes. Visualize a simple object in front of you. It can be a cross, or a cube, or whatever you like. I use a silver Ankh for my focus. Visualize the object, until it seems as real as it would if it were really in front of you, and you were seeing it with your eyes open.

7. Once the object is solid in your visualization, start making it revolve around an axis, turning completely around while you watch it. Notice all the details of the object, every curve, and every part of it.

8. Once you have a solid visualization of the moving object, you will also be deep in an Alpha state meditation, and partially into Theta. Replace the object before you with a simple movie screen.

9. Settle back into your mental theater seat. Start eating a bag of mental popcorn. Watch as the scene opens with the beginning of the action of your Persona. Watch as he or she follows the script that you made for doing the action that you plotted out, for you to follow. At any time during the show, you can stop and start the movie at any place.

10. When you have finished watching the movie, you can watch it again. You can also sit in a comfortable and deep meditation, and let all your tensions flow away.

11. When you finish, and open your eyes, know that you are that person you just watched. Make a special effort to react to everything that happens the rest of the day as that version of you would. This is a simple version of the Actor's Gambit, where the Actor learns all about the character he is to play. He then becomes that person while reciting the lines. You can always tell when an actor does this. He or she will deliver the lines in a believable manner.

12. Every morning and every night, you will find a few minutes to read a set of affirmations of the person you are. The new Persona is the you that you are affirming.

13. You will be well acquainted by this time with the ways that your new self will react to situations. Think about this new and better set of habits of behavior and thought. Try every time you take an action to repeat these same habits.

14. From now on, as soon as you have decided on a course of action, you will begin working on it immediately. You recognize that taking any action toward your goals is far better than doing nothing. By now you must realize that when something does not work, you should do something different, and do it now!

15. Now we have reached the final item on this list. Every morning when you get up, make a point to 'put on' the new Persona, mentally, just like you would put on your clothes. Make a point throughout the day to remember that you are wearing the new You.

# 15: GOAL STEPPING

**We** have covered most of the parts of a life plan to get your goals. It will work for any goal you might have, but we will follow the process through for the loss of weight. We know that a large part of the goal of losing weight will be to change your diet. I expect you to start immediately researching various sources of information dealing with the Paleo Diet online.

As you compile a list of useful websites for your goal, I expect you will also be changing your grocery list to get the correct ingredients. You can work the steps of the plan to lose the weight while you do this.

First, you defined the goal and wrote it down. It goes something like this:

**I will weigh 120 pounds by the end of 2016. I will maintain that weight for the rest of my life. It will be a healthy, enjoyable process of seeking and getting an unending list of goals I desire in life.**

You rewrote this goal as an affirmation:

**I am at my perfect weight of 120 pounds. I am happy, creative, and successful in every activity to which I turn my attention. Life is better for me every day.**

You have decided which beliefs you had that would benefit you. You know which ones were bad for you. You know which new ones you need to have:

**I believe that I have a destiny.**

**I believe that I deserve to be happy, and have, do, or be anything I wish to be.**

**I believe that I can do anything I set my mind to doing.**

**I believe that I create the world I inhabit. I trust myself to create a better world.**

**I believe that I can be, and I deserve to be slender, healthy, and happy.**

You have described the new YOU that will be your consciously created Persona:

When I look in the mirror, I see:

**-An ME that weighs 120 pounds.**

**-I am attractive, happy, and creative.**

**-Creates my world, not controlled by it.**

You have described a place where you can live within your mind. There, the power of your mind to create your world is pure and unlimited. There you are absolutely safe and comfortable. This is your Mind Palace.

You have described a short mental movie. This movie shows the new YOU performing actions successfully toward the weight issue.

You sat down in a private, comfortable place. You close your eyes and visualized the new YOU in the middle of your Mind Palace. You drew energy up from the Earth, and Down from the sky. You let it wash through you and heal you.

When you are relaxed, you started visualizing a focus object of your choice before you. When you can see it consistently as though you see it through your eyes, you start rotating it before you. You see every detail of the object as it turns.

When the rotating Focus is clearly and consistently seen, dismiss it. Now see a movie screen before you. Start the movie that you have prepared. See YOU accomplishing the action that you wrote for the movie.

Repeat the movie, or just meditate while the energy washes you clean. When you decide to end the meditation, recite the affirmation to yourself. See the new YOU when you see yourself. Start the next step toward the goal of losing the weight.

Try consistently to BE the YOU that you have designed the rest of the day. You know the character. Always act *as if* you are the new Persona.

Repeat the meditation and visualization process every morning when you awake. Repeat it every night before you sleep.

End each meditation with the affirmation.

Each morning, after you have meditated, mentally 'Put On' your new Persona. Wear it all day long.

You have worked out a proper menu to eat. You have learned to eat small meals very slowly. You realize that your life can be so engaging and active that you are more likely to forget to eat than to overeat. You have determined the minerals and vitamins, which the foods you have bought are lacking. You have secured them in supplement form.

You have made a list of tasks to do to complete and maintain the physical side of the goal. They are priority ranked on the list. Take the highest priority items from the list and put them on a simple TO-DO list.

As soon as you completed your daily morning tasks, such as eating and brushing your teeth, you go out and do the items on your list. Do this every day as long as physical actions exist to take toward the goal.

Repeat this routine every day, until the habits, beliefs, expectations, and self-image of the new Persona are the only ones that still exist within you.

# 16: THE PLAN

**Let** us recap our progress so far. You have decided that you will eat a well-balanced menu every day. You will supplement for your food deficiencies in minerals and vitamins. You will eat several small meals a day instead of the standard three. You will eat each one very slowly.

You have picked the primary goal of weight loss. You have picked two secondary goals. You wrote out each of them and put the two secondary goals away. You have now rewritten the primary goal as an affirmation.

You have picked the beliefs that would benefit you in getting your primary and secondary goals. You realized which negative goals you had, and decided to get rid of them in your new Persona. You wrote down your new set of beliefs that would be helpful for you to hold.

You have imagined the perfect place for you to be when you are working on your goals. It is a place where you are safe, comfortable, and happy. This will be your Mind Palace.

You have imagined and constructed you new Persona. You will wear this Persona when you are working on all your goals, in the future. This new Persona will be your new personality. You will be working on your goals all the time.

You imagined the new Persona. You can describe every aspect of the Personas appearance and behavior. You find yourself daydreaming about yourself as the Persona, as you are going about your day.

You wrote out a full description of the new Persona. You have also made a point of seeing those new characteristics that the Persona has, every time you look into the mirror.

You have written out the plot of your new Persona acting to get the goal. You sat down and essentially wrote out a screenplay of the new mental movie that you will watch.

You sat down in a secluded and comfortable place and closed your eyes. You see your Mind Palace all around you. You visualized a simple object in front of you. This is your focus object. You study every part of the object until it seems real to you. You then start it rotating before you. You visualize it in every detail.

As you watch the focus, rotating before you, you see and feel the energy coming down from the sky, or ceiling, and coming up from the ground, or floor. The energy looks like lightning, or just as light, and as it enters you, it calms and energizes you. The energy flows through you, cleansing your body and mind of toxins of all kinds, and healing any diseases or injuries that exist.

As you watch the focus, and feel the energy move around, into, and through you, you become more and more relaxed. You are now in a deep meditative state. When you feel ready, you dismiss the focus before you. You visualize a simple movie screen.

You are totally calm, and comfortable, and in deep meditation. The movie that you have created begins, and you see the new YOU on the screen. You see yourself slender and healthy. You see YOU going through a day where you are happy and eating right. You are actively pursuing your every desire. No place exists in this life for being overweight.

The movie rolls on to the end. As the ending credits start, you start coming up out of the meditative state. You make it a habit of doing this same meditation, with the mental movie, every day.

As you come out of the meditation, you 'Put On' the Persona. You rise from the chair. You spend the rest of the day as the Persona. You know all about how Actors assume the personality of a new character. You make a point of doing the same exercise. You use the Actor's Gambit to shore up any problems with the new YOU.

As soon as you are out of the meditation, you immediately start working on the next item on the To-Do list that you carry around to accomplish your goals.

The Plan is simple. It is also a bit repetitious, but it will work if you work it. If you think about it, this is a universal constant. Most of the things you do to get important things are simple acts. Carrying them out will get you what you want.

Do not abandon your exercises. Do them every day, and when you have the goal accomplished that you were working on, maintain it. Immediately start on the next most important goal on your list. This procedure is the one that every successful person uses to get what he or she wants.

# 17: INFINITE LIFE

**I** don't *know* you. You may be well on your way to putting all the procedures in this book to work for you, or you may not have done a thing. Life is all about *choosing* your actions. You have the right not to change for the better. It is up to you.

The fact is that we make our lives what they are. Our lives can be as limited or as unlimited as we choose to make them. Whether you believe in a spiritual aspect to life, or you are a concrete, non-spiritual person, there are always actions that you can take to make your life better. If you have read this far, it is likely that you spent a lifetime already, making at least part of your life worse than it could be. Is it not the time to change?

It does not matter if you are a New Age type 'looking for the Secret' person, or a no-nonsense Go-Getter, the procedures outlined in this book *can* work for you. While loosely aimed at losing weight, the methods discussed can be used to get anything that you want in life. Is it not the time for a happy life?

The fact is that humans are only happy when they are pursuing their goals in life. Think about it. Just sitting on the couch watching television is a waiting game. It just fills the time until something happens that means something to you. That is a rough definition of happiness.

Happiness is the state of mind that you have when an event happens in line with what you want. You can have all the money in the world and not be happy. If you enjoy accumulating money, the process of getting it can make you happy, but the actions make you happy, not the result.

Even when you have the money, it is not until you use it as a tool to do something that it brings you into a happy state again. Life is not a single event; it is a long series of events. The only end of it is with your last breath.

Just as humans are only happy when pursuing goals, humans are also only healthy when they are happy. If you want to be healthy, you have to live in a way that makes you happy, and that requires you to have goals and to be working on them. Never stop working your goals.

If you are a concrete person, you can approach problem-solving using the same methods that the ancient Hebrews did. If you want to have money all your life, make a rule that you will save 10% of your income always. If you want to eat a healthy diet and avoid diseases, make rules that permit or exclude certain foods.

If you are a more spiritual person, consider the infinite nature of the universe, and accept that anything is possible. Not only are miracles possible, but they are also everywhere. Evidence abounds that the world is full of magick. You have only to open your eyes to see that the universe always brings you what you expect.

There are three broad categories of swords that exist. The Broadsword was a heavy bladed weapon, meant to use against other armored and similarly armed foes, used to hack like an ax and to beat back the foe and his sword.

The second type was the thrusting weapon. You always point the tip at the foe's heart and use the guard to deflect the foe's thrusts. The foil is the lightest of this category of weapon.

The final type is another hacking sword, lighter and more maneuverable than the broadsword. It is meant to be used to cut opponents with the blade that are not armored or similarly armed. It could be used on foot, or on a horse. The saber was the typical example of this type of sword.

We are all like one or more of these kinds of swords. Some of us hack our ways through obstacles, just like a good broadsword. Some of us aim straight at our goals, strategically thrusting to the heart of every problem, like a foil. Many of us are like the saber, slashing at our problems when we approach them.

Life is like a saber. It is curved and unwieldy when it is motionless. It is hard to handle because of the built-in curve to the blade. It becomes poetry in motion when we start to move it toward our goals. Life is meant to be lived, not waited out. Never stop the movement toward what you want.

I hope that you have learned two important lessons by reading this book. If you take no action toward fixing your issues after reading this book, you will be one of the 95% of people that never take advice, whom everyone who ever gave advice knows well. I cannot even tell you with certainty that life is about being happy. I prefer to be happy. The only absolute truth is that life is about living, at least as long as you live it.

Life delivers two different benefits to the Liver. Everyone who lives collects experiences, the good, the bad, and the ugly. Who is to say which of these are more valuable? Another benefit it supplies is information. Whether this comes as data, knowledge or wisdom is also up for debate.

The first lesson this book teaches you is this. You are always what you believe. If you believe yourself to be a Loser, you are. If you think you are a Winner, you are. Whether or not you deserve a reward or a punishment is made real by your beliefs.

When you project your beliefs onto objective reality, it becomes the other side of the belief coin. It becomes an expectation. Your world is entirely made by what you expect it to be. The world you make is entirely up to you.

## THE END

# Also by JD Lovil

## Non-Fiction

Becoming Libertarian
Libertarian Survivalist
Unknown Visitors
Whacking Happiness
The Writer's Plan

## Fiction

Worldship Praxis
Shadow of Worlds
Vanguard of Man
Jigsaw World
The Hand In Shadow

# ABOUT THE AUTHOR

## JD Lovil

Is the writer of a number of cross-genre science fiction novels dealing with the existence of a multitude of parallel earths as required by the Many Worlds interpretation of Quantum Theory. He enjoys writing books which are essentially 'stand alone' books, but with similar rules and circumstances, and with some crossover of characters.

JD also writes nonfiction books occasionally on subjects, which he believes to be given less attention than called for, or for which he perceives a significant need.

Originally from Arkansas, JD Lovil now lives in Phoenix, Arizona.

If you enjoyed this book, please consider leaving a favorable Five Star review at the site where you purchased it. Good reviews are life or death for Authors, and I would really appreciate a good review from you!

You may connect with the Author on Facebook at:

https://www.facebook.com/jd.lovil.9

You may also connect with the Author on Pinterest:

http://www.pinterest.com/jdlovil9

See what he is tweeting about on twitter at:

https://twitter.com/jdlovil

Read on for a preview of

**Unknown Visitors**

Available in the same venue as this book

# CHAPTER 4: ORIGINS

A simple, and at the same time very complex question plagues the mental state of the thinking man today. The answer to that question will determine both the past and the future of our species. That question will either give our lives meaning in the living or take it away. Some of us are not ready for that question. Some of us are. Are you ready to know the question? Here it is.

What are we, and where did we originate? Such a simple two-part question, but it defines all of the purpose and destiny of the human race. Did we evolve, mutation by mutation, unassisted over millions of years, or did an intelligent agency create us, in whole or in part? Are we orphans of the universe, or does our species have parents?

The Reader should be very familiar with the tendency of our species to *need* the existence of an Uber-parental God to show them the way to live. Christians have Yahweh; Muslims have Allah, and so on. It seems that we conspire to find some god to believe in, no matter what our circumstances are. Even Atheists make a god of the non-existence of God, as weird as that seems.

Humans once borrowed a few wolf puppies and proceeded to breed the offspring selectively, until finally, they had the sort of pets and helpmates they were seeking to make. The dogs that the wolves had become accepted humans automatically as their alpha males, leaders of the pack, and as a sort of secondary parent as well.

Modern dogs *need* humans in their lives. Even the most feral dogs have a noticeable depressive state going on because they were bred to need the existence of humans in their lives. Imagine a day when suddenly dogs are a little smarter, and humans have vanished from the earth. Would it be unexpected for the dogs to create the *concept* of a beneficent human who watches over them and helps them?

Humans have the same need and concept of a human-like God that people automatically view as superior and beyond challenge, but that brings meaning and all manner of wonderful things to the living. It is obvious to me that not only did *something* have a hand in our development that we saw as a superior human sort of being, but it also made itself fairly indispensable to our psychology.

The question is not if we were designed or modified by some other intelligence. The question is when, why, and how much modification is due to that intelligence, and where are they now? We would also like to know what sort of thing that other intelligence was. Was it some physical entity like ourselves, or was it something more metaphysical, similar to what we consider the big G God to be? Finally, we would like to know why we were created. Were we companions, or Art, or were we supposed to do some task for our creator(s).

To get a handle on these questions, we need to consider the history of our species. When did we come to be, how were we helped, and why, and what information is available to evaluate for accuracy. To know what we are, we have to learn where we came from, and what, if anything, we were designed to do.

Modern science tells us that the human species is no more than 200 thousand years old, using the most liberal of definitions. They would say that the existence of agriculture and animal husbandry occurred about ten thousand years ago, again applying the most liberal of definitions. The concept and construction of cities happened shortly after agriculture became a going concern, and the various monoliths in the world were built shortly after that.

They tell us that the human species is no older than the 200,000 years stated, 'modern' man, maybe less than half as old, civilization dating only to ten millennia ago, with the oldest 'real' civilization being the Egyptian one, maybe four to five thousand years ago.

They neglect to mention that the Sumerian Empire was at least one to two thousand years older than the Egyptians, with the Indus Valley civilization being at least as old as the Egyptian, with records reputed to go back at least ten thousand years or more. They neglect the 200 or so cities found under the ocean, theoretically submerged by the rising waters created by the end of the last glacial age at least ten to eleven thousand years ago.

One interesting factoid about the cities of the Sumer Empire is that they were planned cities, laid out according to a plan that was quite exacting. Planned cities are actually **preplanned**, meaning there was some version of a blueprint created before the city was built. An innovation such as that suggests a good deal of experience in the building of cities. Whoever planned the cities of Ur and Nippur and the rest had done it many times before.

An interesting read that ties Enki, the Anunnaki, ancient city building and a source of ancient knowledge allowing these things to happen is:

http://www.bibliotecapleyades.net/sumer_anunnaki/es p_sumer_annunaki34.htm

Other overviews of sunken and ancient cities are:

http://blog.world-mysteries.com/mystic-places/ancient-cities-and-megalithic-sites-underwater/

http://www.viewzone.com/adamscalendarx.html

http://www.abovetopsecret.com/forum/thread98945/pg1

http://www.abovetopsecret.com/forum/thread657629/pg1

Let us take a moment to reflect on what we (read that as me) are trying to accomplish here. I have deluged you with all manner of alternative information to the standard doctrine of modern disciplines. I am not trying to get you to accept my interpretation of these 'possible' facts. I am not trying to get you to believe any particular point of view.

I am attempting to give you enough food for thought, to show you as many 'what ifs' as it takes to make you question everything you think you know about these subjects. It is my belief that we do not need to have a belief on every subject we consider. It is enough to consider the possibilities.

Maybe the ancient gods were real, physical beings, maybe not. Maybe we were tinkered with by somebody else, maybe not. It is of no value to convince others of a lie. We all need to be open-minded enough to seek the truth without bias.

One thing I can tell you about modern science is that there is a great deal of bias. Modern Archeologists would rather cover up the truth than to give up their pet theories. The Creationists would rather deny evidence than to admit that evolution has its place, and the Evolutionists would rather deny any data that might imply that the development of humanity or any other organism might not be pure evolution.

It is time to introduce some rather interesting information that is strongly influenced by Lloyd Pye. Some of the following information is my interpretation of theories and data from one of his books.

In his book, Lloyd goes through an exhaustive examination of human physiology, genetics and geological and archeological data to support the idea that we were, at least in part, created by extraterrestrial beings. He was a believer in Zacharia Sitchin's Anunnaki theory, and so he believed that the Anunnaki altered humanity to work in the mining of gold for them.

I do not know if Zacharia's theory was true, so I do not know whether the Anunnaki altered Man for that purpose, but Lloyd certainly did his homework. Here is a brief run-down of what he thought.

He notes that the gold mines indicated existed in the same area of Africa where humankind supposedly evolved. He notes that the foot, leg, and hip of humans are not optimized for walking in the manner in which he walks, while most animals evolve a much more efficient locomotion method during the evolutionary process.

He noted that Homo Sapiens, and presumably the previous Hominids, possess 23 pairs of chromosomes, while the primates possess 24. He notes that one of the chromosomes of Man is a combination of two of the original chromosome, somehow glued together by methods unknown.

He noted that our genetic ancestry is 97-99 percent the same as the primates, indicating that we are indeed related, but we have a number of unusual genes that are not part of their genome.

He defines a difference between the primates, which are all of the monkey varieties, the Hominids, which includes Man, Neanderthal and all of the ancestral forms that we all know and love, and the Hominoids, which is the Big Foot, Sasquatch, and various other types of manlike creatures that have an unknown relationship to our species.

I would like to redefine these slightly. The Primates are the 24 pair of chromosomes set consisting of the monkeys and the great apes. The Hominids are the species that are associated with our evolution into Homo Sapiens from the common ancestor. The Hominoids are anything else that has a form similar to that of Man but are not Man.

I would say that Big Foot could actually be a Hominid. We do not know. Call him hominoid until we know different. Add in every described alien visitor that we know of, current and historical. We cannot verify that a Reptilian is in any way related to us, but it is bipedal, and it walks in a way that screams either Hominid or Hominoid.

Maybe I am wrong. Maybe aliens are real, but everything we have ever seen is a robot operated by remote control by tentacled alien starfish. Nobody knows, but let us call a spade a spade, at least until we discover that it is actually a pitchfork.

Let us return to our narrative. The speculative theory that we are exploring is that aliens landed on earth, possibly to mine gold, modified a hominid they found here for unknown reasons, possibly to assist them, and over time gave us knowledge that helped us build cities, grow food and look at the heavens in wonder.

There are monoliths that have been discovered which we could not build with our current standard building equipment. We have to ask ourselves two questions regarding this. First, *how* did they build them with the primitive tech that we have assumed, and secondly, *why* would they build them instead of devoting the energy to survival?

These are not idle questions. Nowhere in the world has there been a building project on such a massive scale in historical (non-god directed) times, because they are never so rich that they can afford the effort. Such a misuse of energy would lead them to famine and destruction.

If one drops pre-conceived ideas about history, a couple of possibilities suggest themselves. Perhaps the gods were real, and they were the builders of these massive structures. Perhaps the gods had taught humankind how to do the construction, and it was humans using very advanced technology to complete the projects. Perhaps it was all human derived, but the technology was from an older human civilization, used to build the structure, and later lost.

There are probably a number of other possibilities, but these will do for now. Let us assume the Anunnaki were real, and lived here on earth, and created, or at least tweaked humanity. I still have a part of the story that bothers me.

If the Anunnaki created Man, what was the purpose of creating a creature so close to themselves in looks and actions? This would lead to a very complicated relationship with these slaves. Even the gods must have found it difficult not to empathize with beings so similar to themselves. Did that not make it hard to treat humanity as the tool it was supposed to be?

Engineering and dealing with biological slaves has to be

much harder than dealing with a programmed, robotic, metal tool. Surely, the Anunnaki had the tech to build an army of robots. Why did they need humanity at all?

As impressive as the technology of the Anunnaki was, it falls far short of what I would expect of a space-faring species with a long history. I would have expected to hear about nanotechnology, some sort of antigravetics or inertial drives. It sounded as though the gods considered rockets, and nukes, to be the height of technology. That would be a little disappointing.

**End of Preview of Unknown Visitors, Chapter Four**

www.ingramcontent.com/pod-product-compliance
Lightning Source LLC
Chambersburg PA
CBHW071407280526
45787CB00001B/472